ANESTHESIA FROM COLONIAL TIMES

A History of Anesthesia at
The University of Pennsylvania

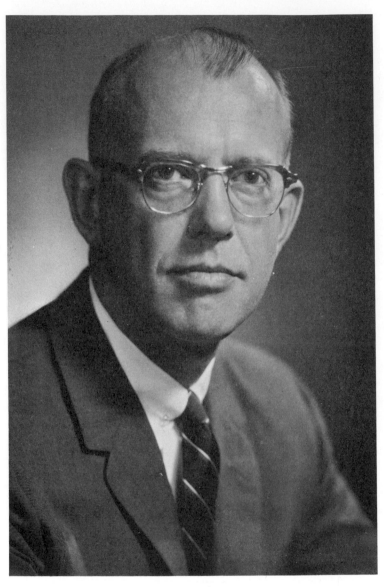

ROBERT D. DRIPPS, MD

ANESTHESIA FROM COLONIAL TIMES

A History of Anesthesia at The University of Pennsylvania

By

JAMES E. ECKENHOFF, BS, MD, FFARCS

PROFESSOR AND CHAIRMAN OF THE DEPARTMENT
OF ANESTHESIA, NORTHWESTERN UNIVERSITY

J. B. LIPPINCOTT COMPANY
Montreal & Philadelphia

Dedication

This History is Dedicated
With Respect and Affection
To a Man Who Has Placed
All Anesthetists in His Debt

ROBERT D. DRIPPS

Foreword

OVER the past century, the attitude of the American medical profession and of surgeons, in particular, toward the pioneers in anesthesia offers an excellent example of what zoologists have called the "instinct of territorial command" and "the pecking order," characteristics which sociologists find also in humans.

This beautifully written and detailed history of the attempts to relieve pain at the University of Pennsylvania shows very clearly the struggle that has been necessary there and in so many other medical schools of this country. In all too many localities, tne "territorial dominance" of the hospital and faculty organization has had to be overcome. At the same time, one has seen the serious frustrations and humiliations suffered by the pioneers during their efforts to bring better methods, drugs, and technics to the service of those patients who come to doctors for the relief of their suffering.

Efforts such as these described at Pennsylvania are overcoming the dominance of anesthesia by nonanesthetists. At the same time, these efforts have eliminated much of the severity of the "pecking" endured by the pioneers. The faculty, the hospital, the surgeon, and the general public from which our patients come, have all benefited in ways just beginning to be appreciated.

As a thorough, workmanlike, and well-documented history of the Department of Anesthesia at the University of Pennsylvania, this monograph will long remain a model for other institutions to emulate. This history will also serve as a well-deserved monument to the labor, enthusiasm and ability of Robert Dripps, who deserves the highest praise, and of his associates.

RALPH M. WATERS
Christmas, 1965

Preface

THE UNIVERSITY OF PENNSYLVANIA School of Medicine celebrated its Bicentennial Anniversary, the first Medical School in the United States so privileged, in 1965.

In this same year, Anesthesia at Pennsylvania gained recognition by being designated an autonomous University department, thus becoming the fifth departmental offspring of that course of instruction given by William Shippen, Professor of Anatomy and Surgery, from 1765 to 1805. And, as the year closed, Robert L. and Grace S. McNeil made a bequest to the University that has led to the creation of the Robert D. Dripps Professorship of Anesthesia.

For these reasons, it has seemed appropriate to take stock, to enumerate the contributions made to anesthesia by Pennsylvania and its faculty, and to document the founding of the present department and its achievements.

JAMES E. ECKENHOFF
1 February, 1966

11

Contents

A History of Anesthesia at
The University of Pennsylvania

I

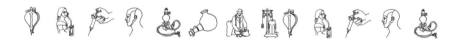

BEFORE SURGICAL ANESTHESIA

LITTLE CAN BE FOUND OF THE METHODS USED TO RELIEVE THE PAIN OF surgical operations at Pennsylvania before the advent of ether anesthesia. However, surgical procedures were not common, and the survivors must not have included writers (see page 19). The earliest mention of presently known anesthetics by a member of the Pennsylvania faculty seems to have been that of Benjamin Rush, Professor of Chemistry on the foundation of the Medical School. Rush was familiar with ether, oxygen and nitrous oxide.[80] In 1801, a syllabus of his Course of Lectures [81] listed "spirits, opium, and ether" under the category of "Internal Stimulants." A search through volumes of notes, recorded by medical students enrolled in Rush's courses, does not suggest a significant discussion of ether, yet infrequent pertinent statements are found. In one volume,[79] the following was written during a lecture on colic: "Ether a sovereign remedy in the cholick"; for the treatment of pertussis, "Inhalation of oxygene gas diluted with atmospheric"; and for the treatment of asthma, "Remedies————, ether ————, skunk oil, ————, oxygene gas" (the blanks were not decipherable). In another volume,[93] the notes indicate that Rush said that ether is given by way of the lungs, and that "In prostration by malignant fever loud noises be avoided and initially ether and ardent spirits." Finally, Rush raised the following question about relieving artificial pain: "Might we not induce coma to a low degree of apoplexy in order to bear long operations and parturition well?" None of these notes makes direct reference to nitrous oxide, but it is apparent that he was aware of the gas.

In 1794, Philadelphia was swept by an epidemic of yellow fever, during which Pennsylvania lost its Professor of Chemistry. Joseph Priestley, one of the discoverers of oxygen and of nitrous oxide, came to America just at that time, seeking political and religious freedom. He was offered the vacant professorship, but declined, writing [13] that at first he wanted to accept because the faculty appointment would allow him to form a Unitarian congregation in Philadelphia, but when he realized that four months of every year would have to be spent away from home, he declined. Had his books and apparatus been in Philadelphia, he said, he might have acted differently. He spent the remainder of his life in Northumberland, a hundred miles from Philadelphia, and remained in close touch with the medical faculty.

After Priestley's rejection, James Woodhouse was appointed, and became the most brilliant American chemist of his generation.[88] Woodhouse did more than anyone except Lavoisier to establish proof of the existence of oxygen, by disproving the phlogiston theory that had kept Priestley from making the most of his original observation on "dephlogisticated air." [88] He conducted elaborate experiments before large classes of medical students, demonstrating theories and chemical actions. He knew of Priestley's discovery of nitrous oxide, and also of Humphrey Davy's investigations with that gas. Woodhouse would prepare nitrous oxide and invite a few students to breathe it with the

16

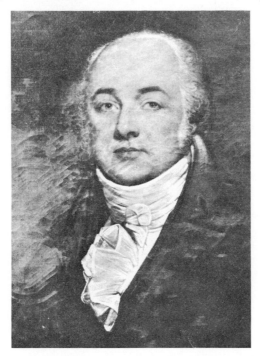

FIGURE 1. *Portrait of* JAMES WOODHOUSE, *Professor of Chemistry 1795–1809, painted by Rembrandt Peale.* (Reproduced with the permission of the College of Physicians, Philadelphia.)

remainder as witnesses (Figure 1). The volunteers usually were "exhilarated." [8, 88] For a time, Woodhouse doubted the cerebral effects of nitrous oxide. One day, he had believed the nitrous oxide that he had prepared impure, released it, and refilled the container with atmospheric air. He did not notify the students of the change, and when they breathed the gas, he observed that their responses were much the same as those usually seen when nitrous oxide was breathed. This forced him to the conclusion that the effects of nitrous oxide were imaginary. It was years later before he became convinced that nitrous oxide did affect the mind. One may speculate that more might have come of this work had Woodhouse not died from overwork in 1809.

Among the students witnessing these demonstrations were Benjamin Silliman and W. P. C. Barton. Silliman, revered as the founder of the

17

Medical School at Yale University, was appointed Professor of Chemistry and Natural History at Yale without special knowledge of the field. He studied with Woodhouse in 1803–1804, and continued the demonstrations of nitrous oxide on his students in New England.[87] Barton, later a Professor of Botany at the University of Pennsylvania and Professor of Materia Medica at Jefferson Medical College, was especially intrigued with nitrous oxide and, with Rush's assistance,

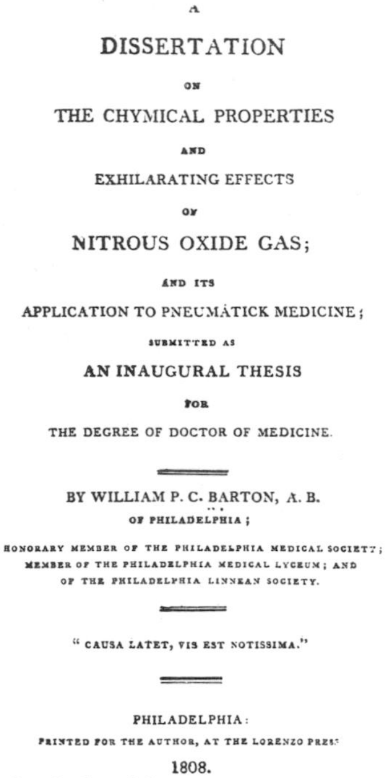

A

DISSERTATION

ON

THE CHYMICAL PROPERTIES

AND

EXHILARATING EFFECTS

OF

NITROUS OXIDE GAS;

AND ITS

APPLICATION TO PNEUMATICK MEDICINE;

SUBMITTED AS

AN INAUGURAL THESIS

FOR

THE DEGREE OF DOCTOR OF MEDICINE.

BY WILLIAM P. C. BARTON, A. B.

OF PHILADELPHIA ;

HONORARY MEMBER OF THE PHILADELPHIA MEDICAL SOCIETY;
MEMBER OF THE PHILADELPHIA MEDICAL LYCEUM; AND
OF THE PHILADELPHIA LINNEAN SOCIETY.

" CAUSA LATET, VIS EST NOTISSIMA."

PHILADELPHIA:
PRINTED FOR THE AUTHOR, AT THE LORENZO PRESS
1808.

FIGURE 2. *Photograph of the title page of W. P. C. Barton's* Dissertation on Nitrous Oxide, *published in 1808.*[8]

experimented with the gas. In 1808, he published a thesis [8] entitled *A Dissertation on the Chymical Properties and Exhilarating Effects of Nitrous Oxide Gas. . .* (Figure 2), containing many observations similar to those of Davy.[24] He wrote that he once inhaled the gas when "I had been affected with vertigo, acute and painful hemicrania, and considerable nausea, induced by a violent blow which I had received upon my head. . . ." As the result of this experience, he said, "I am

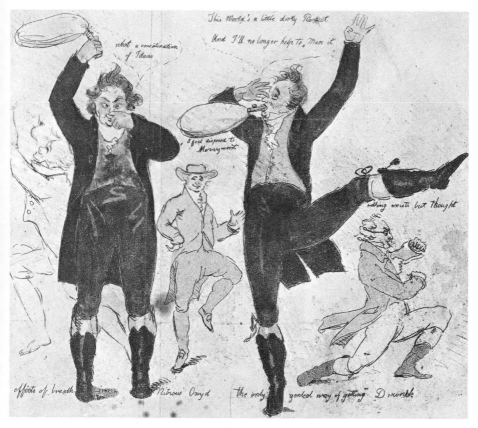

FIGURE 3. *Caricature published in 1808 satirizing the work and thoughts of W. P. C. Barton on Nitrous Oxide.* (Reproduced with the permission of the Edgar Fahs Smith Memorial Collection, University of Pennsylvania.)

decidedly of opinion with Mr. Davy, that this gas has the power of removing intense physical pain." In his thesis, Barton explained Woodhouse's confusion, caused by the sensations experienced by students breathing atmospheric air from closed containers. Carbon dioxide accumulation was responsible. Barton conceived nitrous oxide of use in inhalation therapy, for the treatment of mental disease and for its exhilarating effect (Figure 3). This interest in nitrous oxide was not pursued, although, following the publication of his thesis, he became the recognized authority on the subject.[67]

19

Two further notes come from the pen of George Bacon Wood, who graduated from Pennsylvania in 1818 and later became Professor of the Theory and Practice of Medicine. In his *Treatise on Therapeutics and Pharmacology*, published in 1856,[101] we find: "More that 30 years ago, I remember well that it was quite a fashion among the boys in Philadelphia to inhale ether for its intoxicating effect, which resembled that produced by nitrous oxide. . . . One case of death with coma occurred and several other cases of an alarming character, and the practice soon ceased." He also noted that Phillip Syng Physick, Professor of Surgery 1805–1818, used ether for pulmonary afflictions and had invented a small inhaler for the purpose. Neither Physick's

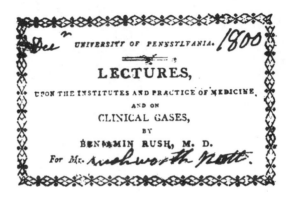

FIGURE 4. *Photograph of a card of admission to the lectures of Benjamin Rush, issued in December, 1800.*

bibliography nor several volumes of lecture notes by his students give further evidence.

All of the academic successors to Woodhouse and Rush wrote of nitrous oxide, ether and oxygen.[44, 23, 19, 101, 102] "Pneumatic medicine" was popular, and a variety of substances, volatile and gaseous, were inhaled for pulmonary diseases. Rush was a leader in this movement (Figure 4), although he does not appear to have written about it.[22] Barton's application of nitrous oxide was toward pneumatic medicine, but one cannot find a serious attempt to apply this to patients. The clinical application of ether before the advent of surgical anesthesia is perhaps best described, in 1831, by Chapman in his *Elements of Therapeutics*: [19]

20

Ether is an active stimulant and antispasmodic, somewhat analogous to alcohol in its leading effects, though more powerful and less permanent . . . its impressions are so evanescent that little is gained by it, and it is difficult to imagine a case in which it should supersede wine, etc.

All references seem to have been to medical patients; what did the surgical patient experience during an operation before the days of

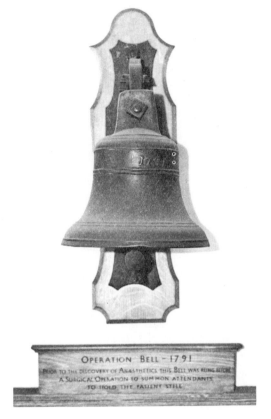

Figure 5. *Operation Bell, 1791. A poignant recollection of surgical procedures before the days of anesthesia. The caption reads:* "Prior to the Discovery of Anaesthetics this Bell was rung before a Surgical Operation to summon attendants to hold the patient still." (Reproduced by the permission of Dr. C. P. Fox of the London Hospital, London, England.)

surgical anesthesia? (See Figure 5.) John Ashhurst, Professor of Surgery (1889–1899), has given a vivid account.[5]

It is difficult to obtain an accurate picture of preanesthetic surgery from the patient's point of view, probably for a similar reason to that indicated by the lion in the fable, when he criticized the artist for always representing a combat between lion and man terminating in a human victory,—lions do not paint; and so as operations are habitually reported by surgeons and not by patients, we read of the skill and intrepidity of the operator, of difficulties met and overcome, and of victories snatched, as it were, from the very jaws of impending defeat; but we hear little of the tortures of the victim under the life-saving process, or, in an unsuccessful case, of the gradual subsidence of agonizing cries hushed in the silence of death.

II

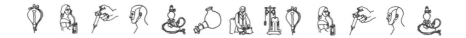

OPPORTUNITY MISSED

OF CRAWFORD LONG, SURELY SOMETHING SHOULD BE SAID, BECAUSE Pennsylvania histories have avoided the subject.[17, 21] In Corner's recent *Two Centuries of Medicine*,[21] an historical account of the School of Medicine, Long's name is omitted, amazingly, and indeed short shrift is given to the entire field of anesthesia. This is a serious oversight, for surgical anesthesia is the major medical contribution of America to the world, and a Pennsylvania graduate figured prominently in its story.[12, 53, 95, 121]

Long was graduated in 1839. Among his professors were George Wood, Hare and Chapman, all of whom wrote and spoke of nitrous oxide and ether. How often Long saw ether used is unknown. It was being used on the medical wards of the Pennsylvania and the Philadelphia General Hospitals, where clinical instruction was then given.[19] It has been said that Long was accustomed to student "ether frolics," but Wood's remarks [101] suggest otherwise. Actually, Long may not have seen much need for surgical anesthesia, if the experience at the Massachusetts General Hospital is typical. In 1846,[50] only 37 operations were performed there. That the faculty "had [its] share in the accumulation of the facts and in the formation of the atmosphere that jointly led to the use of ether in surgery" there can be no doubt.[58] To quote, further, J. William White, Professor of Surgery at Pennsylvania (1899–1919):

. . . when Dr. Long came to us, the reputation of the School had so extended, that our Alumni . . . were filling the most important chairs in the chief medical colleges of the country, two at Harvard, two in New York, two in Winchester, Virginia, two in Lexington, Kentucky, four in Baltimore, six in Charleston, and, as has always been the case, some of our very best with our younger sister, the Jefferson Medical College. There were then 18 medical journals in America, and 10 of them were originated and edited by our graduates. With almost no exception the systematic treatises then in use in Medicine, Surgery, Obstetrics, Materia Medica and Therapeutics had been written by our professors.[58]

When, after graduating and establishing a country practice in Jefferson, Georgia, Long was asked by a group of young men seeking a new experience to prepare nitrous oxide for them to inhale, he answered that the apparatus was not available, but that he did have ether, which would produce the same effect. Presumably, many ether frolics were held before Long excised James Venable's tumor. The patient had been a member of the frolic group and was familiar with the sensations of inhaling ether, so it was natural that he volunteer.

Not until Morton's public demonstration in late 1846, and after the urging of others, were Long's experiences reported, in 1852.[12] Numerous explanations have accounted for this delay, including those of insufficient opportunities to do more cases, unavailability of a suitable patient for a "capital" operation, and local disapproval of the "powers" that Long was demonstrating. Another was suggested by DaCosta, Professor of Surgery at Jefferson Medical College in 1912: [58] "George B. Wood's condemnation of the premature reporting of cases of drug actions. . . ." Perhaps all are correct, although an aggressive personality would have surmounted these obstacles.

One is forced to conclude that Long did not appreciate what he had done. His knowledge of substances with anesthetic potential was no more than that of his professors. He had gone but a short step further in removing a subcutaneous tumor during ether inhalation when he knew trauma would be painless under the same circumstances. Davy, Beddoes, Priestley, Woodhouse, Barton, Hare, Coxe, Chapman and

23

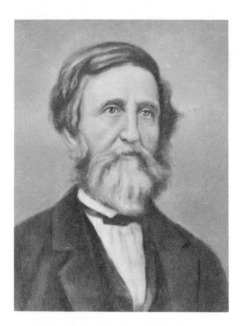

FIGURE 6. *Portrait of* CRAWFORD W. LONG *by Richard Lahey. The painting now hangs near the Medical Library in the Medical Laboratories on Hamilton Walk.* (Reproduced by permission of the University of Pennsylvania).

Wood all knew about nitrous oxide, ether, or both; George Wood taught Long about ether, and he has been described as "an unrivaled teacher in the United States and unsurpassed anywhere." [52] Some of the most brilliant minds of the early nineteenth century held this discovery within their grasp, but all failed to exploit it.

There should be neither surprise nor excuses that Long, too, failed. Perhaps the final suggestion of Long's indifference to the matter is that he never made any effort to claim priority; his part was taken by interested friends or relatives. He, too, was the only one of the four concerned with the ether controversy who led a normal life after 1846; the other three died harassed and demented. The world is filled with superior physicians who disdain publication or podium. Likewise, it has its share of those who would do well to emulate Long's

24

reticence to speak or write and his calm response to the tumult that rose about him (Figure 6).

III

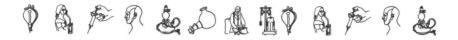

THE FIRST YEARS AFTER ETHER

TO MOST PHYSICIANS IN THE UNITED STATES, SURGICAL ANESTHESIA AROUSED a flurry of interest and controversy, and then subsided into oblivion for half a century. In a measure, this statement is correct, and from its explanation come answers to current problems. With the exception of Long, the men involved in the early demonstration of surgical anesthesia were not physicians. In addition, ether augmented respiration, generally stimulated the circulation, and was an effective analgesic without requiring deep anesthesia. The open-drop or ether-cone technics predominated. Duncum has written [28]

These principles of anaesthetic technic, the rejection of all but the simplest utensils . . . had not only the sanction of intellectual leaders in the old-established medical centers of the Eastern States, but the approval of men practicing among the new settlements and advancing frontier posts of the Middle and Western States. For these men, many of whom had received scanty medical training, the tools of their craft necessarily had to be cheap, simple and reasonably foolproof. Ether anaesthesia appeared admirably to conform to such requirements. That anaesthesia could be looked upon as a science needing an expert to apply it clinically was, to the average American, either unthinkable or ridiculous. In American hospitals so foolproof was etherization considered that it was entrusted to a nurse, or more often still, it was one of the less interesting routine duties to which junior medical students were relegated.

This situation differed from that in England. There, chloroform quickly superseded ether. Its champion, Sir James Y. Simpson, was

25

an eminent physician, and his work stimulated that of others of equal ability. John Snow became the leader of British anesthesia, followed by Clover, Hewitt and Buxton. Chloroform was a dangerous agent and, unless given with skill, death could result. Indeed, death did occur so commonly and in such trivial operations as finally to discredit the agent. However, by then the administration of anesthetics by physicians had been secured.

Concerning the early use of surgical anesthesia in Philadelphia, little is written. Medical students were still being trained at the Pennsylvania or Philadelphia General Hospitals; the University Hospital, the first such institution exclusively for teaching purposes, did not open its doors until 1874. The exact date of the first ether anesthesia in Philadelphia is unknown. Packard relates the following story: [66]

Some years ago a search was made of the records of the Pennsylvania Hospital to see if any account of the first use of ether could be found. The effort was unsuccessful, but Dr. James Darrach of Germantown, who had been resident physician in the hospital in 1846-1847 was still living. He said he could tell about a case which was one of the first, if not the first, in which ether was administered in the hospital. A man was brought in with a crushed leg, which Dr. George W. Norris was going to amputate. Dr. Norris told young Darrach to get some sulphuric ether, saying, "We will try what they are doing up in Boston." Neither Dr. Norris nor Dr. Darrach had ever seen it used but young Darrach poured some on a towel and bade the patient breathe it in. In a few minutes the man became unconscious and, very much alarmed, Darrach called out, "Dr. Norris, the patient is unconscious!" Dr. Norris yelled back at him to "take that damned stuff away!"

Agnew [2] credits Edward Peace, a lecturer in surgery, to have used ether first at the Pennsylvania Hospital, for reduction of a dislocated shoulder. According to tables published in the 1848 *Transactions of the American Medical Association*,[123] the first ether anesthesia for an operation in the Clinic of the University of Pennsylvania was on October 20, 1847, for the treatment of a fissure in ano and the surgeon was "Dr. Horner." This presumably was William E. Horner, Professor of Anatomy 1831-1853, who was also a skillful surgeon and along with Gibson, Professor of Surgery, at that time performed surgical operations at the Almshouse (Philadelphia General Hospital). The second operation with ether anesthesia was on October 27, was listed as an amputation, and the surgeon was again Dr. Horner.

26

Several months did elapse between the October, 1846, demonstration in Boston and the use of ether in either New York or Philadelphia. Again referring to the 1848 *Transactions*,[123] ether was first used in the New York Hospital on February 13, 1847, and at Jefferson Medical College on July 19, 1847. But by the beginning of 1847, many patients had been anesthetized in London. It suggests an incredulous attitude in America. Stillé, Professor of Theory and Practice of Medicine (1864–1884), explains: [91]

This hesitation to accept the new discovery is in some degree attributable to the taint of charlatanism which at first attached to it; to the endeavor to preserve it as a secret; to the title of 'Letheon' with which the ether employed in the first operation was decorated; and to the disgraceful attempt of those who introduced it into surgical practice to obtain a patent-right for their discovery.

There was an early resistance to the use of ether, and some claimed that anesthesia increased surgical mortality. In this instance, a note written in 1848 in a Syllabus of George Wood's Lectures is illuminating: [100] "Dr. Wood thinks that if he were to have a large operation performed he should use this ether." One of the biggest controversies concerned the use of anesthesia in the parturient. Again, to quote Stillé: [91]

Strange though it may now appear, the use of ether was at first strongly reprobated, both in England and in this country, upon the ground that it was sinful to prevent a suffering which had been laid as punishment upon the mother of mankind and her daughters. The objection was produced in so many quarters as to be thought worthy of refutation by good and learned men. At this day it can only be remembered as one of the hallucinations from which the wisest of mankind are not at all times nor ever wholly exempt.

Meigs, Professor of Midwifery at Jefferson Medical College (1841–1861), was markedly antagonistic to anesthesia in obstetrics, as noted by S. Weir Mitchell while a student at Jefferson in the late 1840's: [15]

My father first in Philadelphia used ether in childbed. Professor Meigs violently opposed it and one day undertook to show its peril to a class of three hundred or more at the Jefferson Medical School. A big billy goat was brought into the arena, which was called the bull ring, and Ellerolie Wallace, Dr. Meig's assistant, gave the ether. At last, Professor Meigs

27

announced the demise of Billy, and the corpse was taken out and left in a small room at the half-way landing of the main stairway. The lecture over, we were noisily descending to the chemical lecture when Wallace opened the door to Billy's room. Out came Billy, very drunk, charged between Wallace's long legs into a mass of delighted students, and Billy and students went downstairs in one wild confusion. My father was never weary of inquiring of his colleague after this patient's health.

Despite this experience, Meigs retained his beliefs. Hodge, Professor of Midwifery at Pennsylvania (1835–1869), wrote in 1866: [48]

Professor Meigs has strong protests against anaesthesia in labor, declaring that it is fraught with danger and predicting that, in the course of a few years, it will be banished from practice, except in a few extraordinary cases.

Hodge did not share these beliefs, except for normal deliveries in women with strong constitutions.

The first publication related to anesthetics by a member of the Pennsylvania faculty was written by Henry Hartshorne in 1848. It concerned the inhalation and ingestion of ether and chloroform, and concluded that chloroform was a sedative.[46] In 1854, Hartshorne, the first Professor of Hygiene at the University, became incensed when a Philadelphia dentist was convicted of alleged rape during ether anesthesia, apparently the first recorded court case of rape during anesthesia in America. Hartshorne claimed [47] that if the woman perceived what was done, then she was conscious, accordingly retained voluntary motion, and could not, therefore, give valid testimony to the commission of rape upon her person. Hartshorne's brother Edward, an ophthalmologist, wrote a similar defense,[45] as did Stillé's brother Moreton.[92] Edward Hartshorne is remembered as the physician who wrote *The Testimonial of Members of the Medical Profession of Philadelphia in Behalf of William T. G. Morton*,[96] signed by nearly every influential member of the Philadelphia medical community.

Despite this slowness to exploit the new discovery, Philadelphians were well informed of what was happening throughout the world in anesthesia. The immediacy of medical publication exceeded that of today, exemplified by the announcements and critiques appearing in the *American Journal of Medical Sciences*, edited and published quarterly in Philadelphia. The first accounts of the Boston ether demonstration appeared two months later,[98] and within six months there were seven pages of correspondence from England, including a discussion of the impact of surgical anesthesia there.[32] For the next two years, every issue of this journal had an average of 15 pages devoted to anesthesia.

At first, this was factual reporting without critique, as seen from an excerpt from the October, 1847 number: [30]

The introduction of the inhalation of ether as a means of anulling pain, is the most interesting and perhaps important event in the medical history of our time. We had hoped, in the present number of this Journal, to have been enabled to give a full account of the effects of this agent, so as to furnish our readers with the data for determining its exact effects, its precise value as a means of annihilating pain, and to discriminate the cases to which it is applicable. Unhappily the materials for this do not as yet exist. On every point connected with this subject, much diversity of opinion exists, and even reports of experiments are so far at variance that it is impossible to entirely reconcile them. Under these circumstances, all that we can do is to chronicle the principal facts which have been brought to light and leave our readers to draw such deductions as they may feel that these imperfect materials authorize.

There follows an account of 23 reports, lectures and letters from correspondents. Eighteen months after Morton's demonstration, there is a complete and critical review of two monographs on ether, one by surgeon John C. Warren of Boston, and the other by anesthetist John Snow of London.[9] There is also a summary of the *Report of the Board of Trustees of the Massachusetts General Hospital*, January 26, 1848, concerning the controversy between Morton and Jackson.[10]

None of the members of the Pennsylvania faculty wrote authoritatively on anesthesia for ten years after Morton's demonstration. In 1850, William Gibson, Professor of Surgery (1819–1855), published the last of eight editions of his textbook, and ignored anesthesia; but as Samuel Gross, the eminent surgeon at Jefferson Medical College, said, Gibson never caught up with the current advances of surgery. Gibson's successor, Henry H. Smith (1855–1871), devoted a scant three pages to anesthesia in his 1852 text,[89] the superficial nature of which is apparent:

If experience as to its [ether's] power and mode of administration has not yet been gained, let him at once resort to books (of which there are many) or to schools, or even to travel to distant points, until by study and observation he be satisfied freely of its propriety, and enabled yet further to extend the benefits of this admirable agent for the relief of suffering.

If the faculty were not writing about anesthesia during this decade, at least they talked to students about it. Evidence for this can be seen from the subject matter of the students' theses (Table 1). One or

TABLE 1. *Theses of University of Pennsylvania Graduates 1848–1875* [18]

1848	Foster A. Jenkins	*New Anaesthetic Agents*
1848	Armistead N. Wellfard	*Application of Ether to Surgery*
1849	John R. Jameson	*Etherization*
1850	J. Buchanan Whiting	*Anaesthetic Agents as Adapted to Surgery*
1851	John Buford	*Etherization*
1851	John Harvey, Jr.	*Ether*
1853	Charles F. Heney	*Etherization*
1855	S. Nelson Burgess	*Anaesthetics*
1855	Edward H. Horner	*Anaesthetics*
1856	John M. Boyd	*Anaesthesia in Labor*
1856	William N. Coit	*Anaesthesia*
1857	John C. Bragg	*Anaesthesia*
1857	Nathaniel G. Friend	*Anaesthesia in Labor*
1860	Edward Clarke	*Anaesthesia in Surgery*
1860	Robert B. Harris	*Anaesthesia in Parturition*
1860	J. Wesley Thompson	*Anaesthesia*
1862	C. H. Boardman	*De Novo Anaesthetico*
1864	Quincey Van Hummell	*Use of Ether in Obstetrics Practice*
1865	George Gleim, Jr.	*Etherization*
1868	Isaac Minis Hays	*Anesthesia*
1870	Daniel W. Clancey	*Nitrous Oxide*
1872	Milton Keim	*Anaesthesia*
1874	A. Eldridge Carpenter	*Chloroform and Anaesthesia*
1875	William Baker	*Nitrous Oxide*

two students a year selected anesthesia.[18] Unfortunately, these theses were not preserved—they would be an invaluable source of faculty and student opinion of the day. Certainly, the thoughts of student Edward R. Squibb proved important. Squibb graduated from Jefferson Medical College in 1845, spent four years as a Naval surgeon, and returned to Jefferson in 1851 "to rub up." He noted the varying rapidity with which patients were anesthetized with ether. He attributed this to the difference in quality of the ether then available. When he returned to the Navy in 1852, he observed the generally poor quality of drugs dispensed. He obtained permission to establish a laboratory and to prepare pharmaceutical supplies for the Navy. One of his first accom-

30

plishments was to distill ether, and by 1856 he had established the technic that is essentially unaltered today.[11]

IV

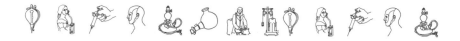

ANESTHESIA AND THE INTERNISTS

THE FIRST DEFINITIVE PUBLICATION CONCERNING ANESTHESIA FROM THE University of Pennsylvania faculty came from the Professor of Medicine, George B. Wood. Fifteen pages of his *Treatise on Therapeutics and Pharmacology or Materia Medica* [101] were devoted to ether, classified as a "Cerebral Stimulant" along with wine and distilled liquor. Chloroform was listed with Cerebral Sedatives, and was allotted 24 pages. The text was critical and interpretative, without documentation. His description of ether analgesia without loss of consciousness is surprisingly similar to that rediscovered by Artusio in 1954: [3]

That ether is capable, when inhaled, of abolishing sensibility, is an obvious corollary to its stupefying powers. The sense of touch as well as every other special sense, is, in the very nature of the case, suspended in coma. This then is no new discovery. But it was not so obvious that the general sensibility might be diminished and even quite suspended, while consciousness, and, to a considerable degree, the special senses, remained unaffected. This, however, is a most important fact in relation to etherization. Under the influence of this agent, pain is often abolished if existing, and averted when it would otherwise have been produced, before the occurrence of any degree of stupor, or of any considerable anesthesia of hearing, sight, etc. The woman in childbed ceases to suffer from her labor pains, though still conscious; the patient under the knife of the surgeon sometimes scarcely suffers, though he may follow every step of the operation.

Wood expressed doubts that ether acted by a chemical effect, since the odor remained on the breath too long after return of consciousness. He viewed the initial excitement and subsequent depression as follow-

31

ing the general law of irritation. He found the thoughts that anesthesia "depraves" the blood and retards healing as nonsense, and pointed out that it was safer than soporific doses of opium. So far as chloroform was concerned, he believed it first affected the cerebral centers of sensation, and as anesthesia deepened, involved the respiratory centers in the medulla and, secondarily, the heart, and finally, the spinal reflex centers and the ganglionic system. He considered chloroform dangerous and to be avoided.

Wood's popular *Treatise* was revised in 1860 and, finally, in 1868. The material concerning ether changed little in the three editions, but increasing space was devoted to chloroform. In all likelihood, this was caused partly by the American concern over chloroform and partly because most of the then current literature originated in Europe and discussed chloroform.

The Professor of Medicine's text continued until 1875 to be Pennsylvania's authoritative work on anesthesia. The surgeon, Smith, had written another text in 1863, and had allotted but five pages to anesthesia, under the heading "Duties of a Surgeon before Operating." It is apparent that questions were being raised about training for the anesthetist, for Smith wrote: [90]

Ether or ether and cloroform mixed in proportion just stated may be safely administered by any well-educated physician. That this is a powerful sedative, and liable to abuse, cannot be doubted; yet it is by no means so dangerous as aconite, morphine, or many other articles of the materia medica in daily use. That any anaesthetic requires to be judiciously or even cautiously administered, is also true, but there is no portion of our professional duties which does not require the same caution; and the liability of anesthetics to be abused is therefore no argument against their proper use.

With all the experience that the Pennsylvania faculty had with nitrous oxide, it is surprising that after the introduction of ether anesthesia, no one reappraised nitrous oxide for surgical anesthesia. The gas was neglected, to lie dormant except as a source of entertainment, until G. Q. Colton, who originally had worked with Wells, again entered the picture. In 1863, Colton was in New Britain, Connecticut, demonstrating to lay audiences the effects of nitrous oxide, when a lady asked if he would administer his gas to her for a dental extraction. He did, the dentist was impressed, and asked to be instructed in the preparation and use of the gas. During the next year, the dentist administered nitrous oxide to over 600 patients,[28] and the use of nitrous oxide for anesthesia was launched.

The next extensive resumé of anesthesia by a Pennsylvanian again came from an internist, Alfred Stillé, who occupied the Chair of Medicine from 1864 to 1884. In the last edition of Stillé's *Therapeutics and Materia Medica*, 74 pages were devoted to ether, chloroform and nitrous oxide.[91] It is obvious that the author did not have personal experience with anesthetics but, rather, presented a compendium of the work of others. Only occasionally did he give his own opinions or summarize those of others, but when he did, he is worth reading. A paragraph suggests that internists did not necessarily see eye to eye with surgeons on the choice of anesthetic agents:

The superiority of chloroform over ether, as a rapid and effectual anaesthetic, caused the latter agent to be in a great measure abandoned by surgeons and accoucheurs in Europe; but the fatal consequences which so often resulted from the employment of chloroform gave a shock to the conscience of the profession, which has led to a more circumspect use of it. We believe that surgeons are more solicitous than they formerly appeared to be to learn, from persons more competent than their special vocation permits them to become, whether the patient is or is not affected with a disease or constitutional peculiarity which should forbid the use of chloroform.

His summation of the existing opinions on the modes of action of nitrous oxide is classic:

If we are to accept these several statements as representing the scientific knowledge upon this subject, we arrive at the following extraordinary conclusions: Nitrous oxide acts primarily upon the heart, and affects the heart last and least of all the organs; it is absorbed into the blood, and is not absorbed at all; it is essentially asphyxiating, yet at one stage of its action essentially exhilarating; it is anaesthetic as undecomposed gas, and only its nitrogen is anaesthetic; the cyanotic hue of the skin is produced by an excess of carbon in the blood, and is due to venous stasis only; and, finally, we may observe that although nitrous oxide is regarded as an anaesthetic by all the other authorities, there are two who maintain that it is not an anaesthetic at all. It may be added that one opinion attributes the exhilaration caused by the gas to the oxygen it contains, although it is well known that oxygen when inhaled produces no such effects, and that exhilarant intoxication is a characteristic effect of the hydrocarbons.

33

Another nationally acclaimed physician at this time contributed to our anesthetic heritage. S. Weir Mitchell, said to be "the most versatile American since Franklin," was graduated from Jefferson Medical College and, although he never occupied a chair at Pennsylvania, he early became a trustee and, subsequently, a Clinical Professor of Neurology.[15] He will be recalled as having first described erythomelalgia.[60] In 1865, he wrote a revealing paper on the antagonism of atropine and morphine,[62] noting, among other things, that atropine always slowed the pulse before increasing it and that atropine and morphine each produced dysuria. These are observations since rediscovered. Mitchell is also remembered for his poem, "Birth and Death of Pain," read at the Ether Semi-Centennial,[61] and as a popular novelist.

V

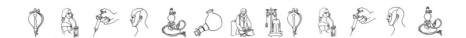

ANESTHESIA AND THE PHARMACOLOGIST

IT WAS ABOUT THIS TIME THAT ONE OF THE NINETEENTH CENTURY'S bright stars in anesthesia appeared. Horatio C. Wood, Sr., nephew of George B. Wood, was graduated from Pennsylvania in 1862, became Clinical Professor of Neurology in 1875 and Professor of Materia Medica in 1876, and held these chairs for 26 and 31 years, respectively (Figure 7). Wood was high strung, somewhat eccentric, energetic, and critical. His first publication related to anesthesia suggested that the search for new anesthetics was in the wrong direction, since it was chiefly among chlorine compounds, which were powerful depressants. He proposed that the ether series be investigated and, with this in mind, reported an investigation on acetic ether, which he found similar to ethyl ether.[104]

In 1874, Wood first published his *Therapeutics, Its Principles and Practice*, a book credited with having done more to put American

34

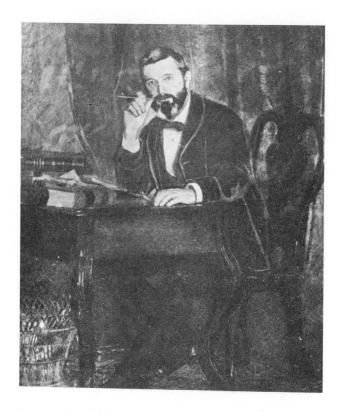

FIGURE 7. *Portrait of* HORATIO C. WOOD *by Thomas Eakins, painted in 1889.* (Reproduced with the permission of the College of Physicians, Philadelphia.)

therapeutics on a scientific basis than any other single work.[106] The text ultimately had 14 editions. The preface of the first edition is apropos today:

At the present time, when the shelves of private and public libraries are groaning beneath their ever-increasing loads, when a thousand presses in every city send forth day and night their printed messages until the earth is filled with them, it seems almost presumptuous for anyone to offer new volumes to the world. Indeed, art is so long, life is so short, that every student has the right to demand of an author by what authority he doeth these things, and to challenge every memoir for its *raison d'etre.* This

35

being so, it assuredly will not appear egotistical for the author to state that his voluntary task was first suggested by his own wants, and that to its performance he has brought the training, labor, and experience of years spent in the laboratory, the study, the classroom, and the hospital ward.

Wood's approach to anesthetics was direct and fresh. Unlike his distinguished uncle, he grouped all anesthetics under a single heading. Differing from Stillé, he devoted only 26 pages to the subject to Stillé's 74, but whereas Stillé required nearly 12 pages to discuss the usefulness of ether and chloroform for nonsurgical purposes, Wood dismissed it in a paragraph. His handling of the theories of narcosis is a delight:

Many of the theories which have been suggested to explain the production of anaesthesia are so groundless that it seems unnecessary to discuss them here. All that are worthy of consideration may, I think, be arranged in four groups, as follows: 1st, those which assert that the symptoms are produced by a partial arrest of oxidation; 2d, those which look upon anaesthesia as due to precedent physical changes in the blood; 3d, those which assert that anaesthesia, like sleep, is due to cerebral anaemia; 4th, those which teach that the various agents employed act directly upon the various organs and tissues concerned,—including in this group the theory of Bernard that anaesthesia is produced by a semi-coagulation of the nervous protoplasm. As the theories of the last group are the most natural, the burden of proof rests upon the supporters of the other theories. All the proofs of the first two groups as yet brought forward amount to no more than as follows: that in profound anaesthesia there is an evident lessening of oxidation; and that some anaesthetics probably produce changes in the blood.

Wood, like all of the other Pennsylvanians, was strong in his condemnation of chloroform anesthesia. He wrote: [106] "So dangerous is chloroform, and so safe is ether, that there is no excuse for the use of the former agent under ordinary circumstances. The reason of the safety of ether is that, unlike chloroform, it does not suddenly paralyze the normal heart." He gathered clinical and experimental evidence for the correctness of his opinions.[117] In 1890, he had a profound influence on the course of anesthesia in Germany, by presenting a paper on Anesthesia at the Tenth International Congress of Medicine in Berlin.[108, 109] The evidence he brought to bear against chloroform was so convincing that it caused German surgeons to survey their own experience, and, within four years, ether had supplanted chloroform in many clinics. Considering the dominant position held by British anesthetists at that time, it is worth noting that this was the second time an American had such an effect on European anesthetic practices.[28] Wood developed contempt for any surgeon who would allow chloroform to be given to his patients.

Interestingly, although Wood pled for more laboratory experimentation, he was unwilling to accept the evidence, provided by the Hyderabad Commission,[97] that chloroform always caused respiratory arrest *before* cardiac arrest. He claimed that the dog environment in India was different from that in America. In 1893, Wood engaged in a spirited debate about the matter with one of his former associates.[110] Hobart Hare had been a co-author with Wood,[42, 117] had done work on chloroform for His Highness, the Nizam of Hyderabad, and in 1891 had been appointed Professor of Therapeutics at Jefferson Medical College. Wood caustically rejected the Hyderabad conclusions, which Hare accepted, and, reverting to published statistics concerning chloroform mortality, said: "If the surgical profession be incapable of observing these simple facts, then I am sorry for those who fall into the hands of the surgical profession."

He pointed out that all anesthetics were potentially lethal:

Anaesthesia will become comparatively safe only when the surgeon recognizes that anaesthesia is an approach to death, and that he ought never give an anaesthetic without recognizing that he is putting the life of the patient in peril and that there is no such thing as a safe anaesthetic.

The discussion that followed was bitter. Hare vigorously defended his position and berated his former mentor. Hare thought poorly trained resident physicians to blame for chloroform's troubles. The audience joined in, divided in sentiments against chloroform. G. G. Davis, later to be Professor of Orthopedic Surgery at the University, said:

In this city the hospitals of the University of Pennsylvania, and I presume the Jefferson, have their official anaesthetizers. Therefore the accidents cannot be attributed to the inexperience of the anaesthetizer except in the other general hospitals.

Hare's rebuttal to this was that hospitals may have their anesthetizers, but that they were usually resident physicians, untrained in anesthetics.

Wood's anesthetic interests were wide and varied. He investigated the use of ethyl chloride and ethyl bromide for general anesthesia [115] and cautioned against their use, his opinions based in part on clinical results obtained in the operating room. He wrote on the treatment of opium poisoning, advising the use of atropine and artificial respiration.[105] He investigated the action of nitrous oxide alone and in combination with oxygen.[111, 114] He studied the action of atropine [119] and alcohol [118] in man, reported on the effects of atropine, strychnine and cocaine on respiration,[116] and examined mixtures of ether, chloroform and benzine for general anesthesia.[113]

Some of Wood's most interesting experiments were published in his excellent chapter on "Anesthesia" in Dennis' *System of Surgery*.[112] This chapter is authoritative not only because of Wood's position in medicine and in the laboratory, but also because of his apparent personal clinical experience. There are no records of how often Wood was an "anesthetizer," but in one article, he wrote: [113]

Especially is there danger of death . . . in the advanced stages of etherization, when the patient is too thoroughly etherized to struggle, and when the attention of the etherizer is, or may be, attracted by some novel and difficult operation. I confess myself to once having nearly killed a patient in this way.

Among the subjects discussed in the chapter are circumstances that modify the choice of anesthetic; preanesthetic medication, wherein he decries the use of large preoperative doses of opium; the after-effects of anesthesia; the technic of administering anesthetics (including the open methods used in America, and the closed or inhaler methods popular in Britain); the importance of skill on the part of the anesthetist; the resuscitation from an overdose of anesthesia. Wood had done a great deal of work on the latter subject, investigating the influence of changes in body position to return blood to a heart nearly paralyzed with chloroform [117] and studying the injectable stimulants then in vogue.[116] These included ether, alcohol, digitalis, strychnine, amyl nitrite and spirits of ammonia. He concluded that amyl nitrite further lowered the blood pressure, alcohol augmented the action of the anesthetic, and ammonia was of little avail, but that digitalis and strychnine were of benefit. Perhaps a fitting concluding quotation from a critical scientist would be his conclusion on the practice of injecting ether hypodermically, to treat an overdose of anesthetic: [116]

Ether in the blood acts as ether, whether it finds entrance through the lungs, through the rectum, or through the cellular tissue; and the man who would inject ether hypodermically into a patient who is dying from ether should, to be logical, also saturate a sponge with the ether and crowd it upon the nose and mouth of his unfortunate victim.

Wood was a prodigious writer. His bibliography contains 273

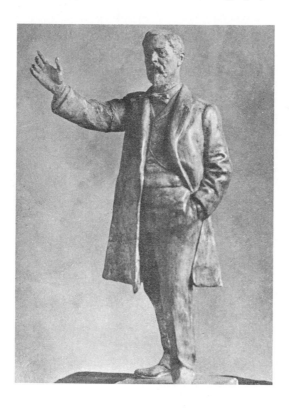

FIGURE 8. *A statuette of* HORATIO C. WOOD *by S. Murray, clearly indicating the character of the Professor in late life.* (Reproduced with the permission of the College of Physicians, Philadelphia.)

publications, at least 17 of which dealt with anesthesia. He died in 1920, leaving a lasting mark upon medicine in America and anesthesia throughout the world (Figure 8).

39

VI

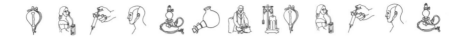

ANESTHESIA AND THE SURGEONS

WOOD WAS THE LAST INTERNIST AT PENNSYLVANIA WHO CONSIDERED anesthesia within his province. But then the surgeons began to think and write more about it. Smith's successor in the Chair of Surgery, D. Hayes Agnew, was a distinguished surgeon [1] and is remembered as the subject of one of Thomas Eakins' famous clinic paintings (Figure 9).

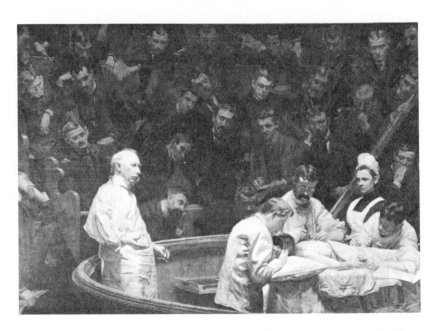

FIGURE 9. THE AGNEW CLINIC, *painted by Thomas Eakins, 1889.*[29] *The painting hangs above the entrance to the Medical Library in the Medical Laboratories on Hamilton Walk* (Reproduced by permission of the University of Pennsylvania.)

40

In this accurate portrayal of a surgical procedure, painted in 1889, an interne is shown administering open-drop ether.[29] Like his predecessors, Agnew wrote a text,[2] including a reasonable although superficial discussion of anesthesia, mostly devoted to safety and technic. He used tracings of pulse waves during ether and chloroform anesthesia to demonstrate the greater safety of ether (Figure 10). John Ash-

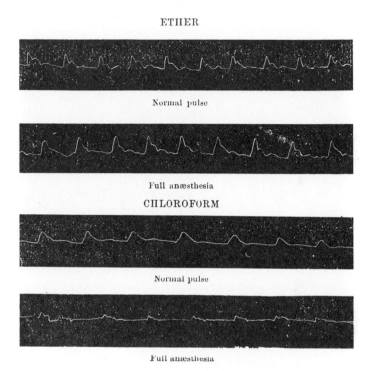

ETHER

Normal pulse

Full anæsthesia

CHLOROFORM

Normal pulse

Full anæsthesia

FIGURE 10. *Reproduction of pulse curves from D. Hayes Agnew's* Text-book on Surgery,[2] *demonstrating the safety of ether as compared with chloroform. The means by which these curves were obtained is unknown.*

hurst, the succeeding Professor (1889–1899), also wrote a text [4] but shunned the task of writing the anesthesia section, turning instead to Henry M. Lyman of the Rush Medical College to do this.[54] Lyman had already established some reputation in anesthesia as the author of *Artificial Anesthesia.*[55]

By the end of the century, a major change in teaching medicine had occurred. Until 1875, instruction was mainly didactic, with fees paid to each professor. In that year, though, emphasis turned to practical instruction and laboratory work, requiring a larger teaching staff. The opening of the University Hospital in 1874 demanded augmentation of the clinical staff as well. Before this time, the faculty was seven professors and a demonstrator in anatomy. In 1880, this had grown to 36 and by 1912 to 270.[21] At present, it is more than 600. With the larger staff and better laboratory facilities, one might have expected more research in anesthetics, but such was not the case. Wood's influence probably accounted for some of the papers appearing before his death. Edward Martin, Professor of Surgery from 1910 to 1918, combined with Hobart Hare, while he was a demonstrator in therapeutics, to investigate the treatment of arrested respiration during anesthesia.[56] This was an anatomical study performed on cada-

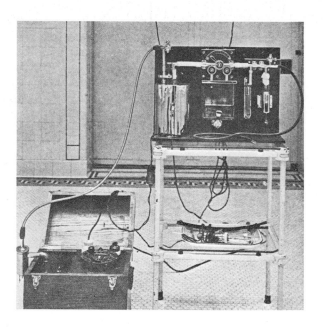

FIGURE 11. *Ether insufflation apparatus in use at the Hospital of the University of Pennsylvania in 1912.* (Photographed from the International Clinics 2 (22nd series), 1912.)

vers, which sought to define the best technic for keeping the airway clear. Another clinical study by Hare [43] documented that body temperature diminished during ether anesthesia. Perhaps this explains the custom of wrapping patients for anesthesia in blankets and applying "ether boots"—a custom very difficult to change. Several individuals [103, 26, 41] were concerned with the influence of ether on the kidneys and urine, and Horatio Wood's son pursued a study, rather superficial, of the effect of small doses of ether and chloroform on sensations in animals.[120]

The remainder of the reports concerning anesthesia by the University faculty were clinical dissertations until the mid 1920's. J. William White, Professor of Surgery (1899–1910), published a lecture on anesthesia,[99] that he had given to students; C. C. Norris compared nitrous oxide with ether anesthesia; [63] and Henry Norris wrote about his experiences with scopolamine-morphine anesthesia.[64] In 1912, Martin and two surgical associates participated in an anesthesia symposium in Philadelphia, which had an international representation (Figure 11).[94]

In 1908 and 1911, two interesting references to cardiac massage were made. The first was found among notes by E. B. Krumbhaar, Professor of Pathology (1932–1948), written when he was a student attending the lectures of J. W. White. The following is quoted from his notebook: [51]

HEART MASSAGE

May be tried in acute failure or syncope, especially if result of anesthetic.

40 cases thus far revived. 9 permanantly. In 8 more, P. and R. returned but patient died later.

3 routes—thoracic, transdiaphragmatic, subdiaphragmatic (best). Has been started after 44 minutes, but no real cure after 7. 30 sec.–5 min. usually enough. Has needed 15. Artif. resp. necessary.

Indications

1. Ac. dilat. in anesthesia, etc.

2. Resp. failure after grad. accum. of chlor.

3. Asphyxia in gen'l.

4. Vital centers stopping from exhaustion or trauma.

Treat

1. Lower head and artif. resp.

43

> 2. *Pressure on abd. aorta, if abd. open, otherwise adrenalin, bandage, Crile suit, NSS.*
> 3. *If unsuccessful start massage—esp. before 1 or 2 min. Continue artif. resp. if neces. for hours.*

The second, by Charles Frazier, Professor of Surgery (1922–1936), was a case report of cardiac arrest with complete recovery.[34] This concerned a 55-year-old male for hydrocelectomy. Difficulty was experienced in establishing ether anesthesia, and chloroform was resorted to. The surgeon was alarmed by the appearance of dark blood in the wound. Cardiac arrest was diagnosed, transabdominal cardiac massage begun with reestablishment of heart action in two minutes, and the operation was completed.

Nearly all Pennsylvanians who have written on anesthesia have ignored Crawford Long. In 1878, Ashhurst wrote that a claim on priority had been made on behalf of Long, but that the evidence in his favor was inconclusive; 18 years later, he repeated the remark.[4] However, in 1912, for the day at least, this was rectified, when a plaque (Figure 12) to Long's memory was dedicated in the Medical Laboratories at Pennsylvania and surgeons from several medical schools spoke in glowing terms of his contribution.[58]

VII

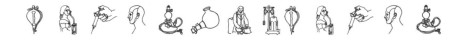

LEADERSHIP LOST

DURING HORATIO WOOD'S TENURE, THE UNIVERSITY OF PENNSYLVANIA WAS the leader in clinical application and in scientific thought in anesthetics in Philadelphia. This status changed at about the time Wood retired. In 1904, W. Wayne Babcock, the celebrated Professor of Surgery at Temple University, learned about spinal anesthesia while visiting Paris. Babcock had expressed concern about anesthetic mortality, com-

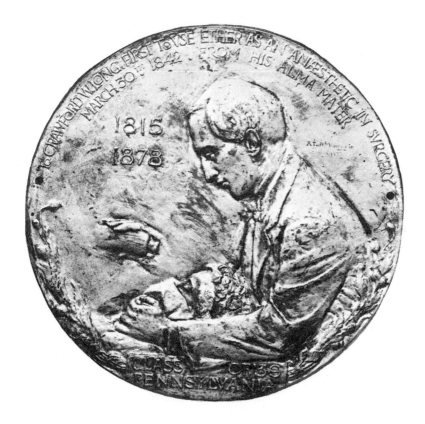

FIGURE 12. *Medallion designed by Professor R. Tait McKenzie, dedicated to the memory of Crawford W. Long on March 30, 1912. The memorial is located near the Medical Library in the Medical Laboratories on Hamilton Walk.* (Reproduced by permission of the University of Pennsylvania.)

menting [6] that although Agnew had written that the mortality from ether anesthesia was 1 in 28,000 administrations, his experience differed. With internes giving ether, he had noted one death in every 500 anesthesias. He became a proponent of spinal anesthesia,[7] believing it safer than general anesthesia, and by 1930 he had published at least 25 papers dealing with this and related technics of anesthesia. During this period, little was heard from Pennsylvania about anesthesia. In 1933, Hahnemann Medical School pushed to the front with the appointment of Henry S. Ruth as Professor and Head of a Department of Anesthesiology, the first such position and departmental status in the city. Hahnemann had had physician anesthetic specialists since 1917, and indeed the first anesthesiologist in the city in Everett A. Tyler. Ruth was trained by Tyler, who administered anesthesia at several Philadelphia hospitals, and was assisted in his early work by two part-time anesthetists-general practitioners, Wayne Killian and James Godfry.* Ruth continued as Professor until his death, in 1956.

While Hahnemann showed foresight in physician-anesthesia specialization, Pennsylvania lagged. It is difficult to be sure who administered anesthetics for the University surgeons until 1938. Before 1874, all of the surgical faculty operated at Pennsylvania Hospital. There, junior resident physicians were usually assigned responsibility for the anesthetic. There is no reason to suspect that this practice changed with the opening of the University Hospital, and in 1889, when Eakins painted the Agnew Clinic, an interne, Elwood Kirby, was portrayed as the anesthetist.[29] Remarks made in 1894 [110] indicated that anesthetics at the University Hospital were given by resident physicians. This was not the rule in the community, as many anesthetics were administered by untrained persons and sometimes, even, by those of questioned intelligence.[16] In 1881, Philadelphia surgeon John Roberts proposed that only trained physicians give anesthetics.[77, 37] In 1908, he made a stronger plea in an article entitled "The Anesthesia Peril in American Hospitals." [78] and proposed a schedule of fees for physician anesthetists. Philadelphia has been credited with having the first full-time physician anesthetist, W. Oakley Hermance, who began practice in 1897 [57] at the Polyclinic Hospital. Unfortunately, this pioneer became disillusioned and changed his specialty to proctology before 1917. At that time, Tyler, who had been in general practice for three years, left the city for anesthetic training with Gwathney, McKesson, Sise,

46

and Bennett, and when he returned he became the only full-time specialist in the city. He retired from practice in 1950 and is living today in Philadelphia.*

* Personal communication, E. A. Tyler.

VIII

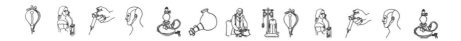

ERA OF THE NURSE ANESTHETIST

JOHN ASHHURST FOLLOWED THE CUSTOM OF HIS CHIEF, AGNEW, IN choosing resident physicians for anesthetists, but White changed things. In 1908, White was operated on at the Mayo Clinic, where he was impressed with his anesthetic, which was administered by a nurse. On his return to Philadelphia, he petitioned the University Hospital Board for permission to appoint and train a nurse anesthetist.* The Minutes of the Executive Committee of the Board of Managers, December, 1908,[59a] contains the notation:

A communication was received from Dr. White, Senior Surgeon, in regard to the appointment of a salaried anaesthetizer. The secretary was directed to inform Dr. White that the matter was already in the hands of the Chairman of the Committee on Medical Affairs for consideration.

No record can be found of approval of the petition, but in January, 1909, a copy of "Rules for the Hospital Anesthetizer" is appended to the minutes. These state that the salary should not exceed $60 monthly, that visiting surgeons would be charged $10 for the anesthetizer's services, while other surgeons would pay $5 to the hospital. The duties outlined were, "to administer the anesthetic." White assigned his surgical assistants, Frazier, Muller, and Thomas to select and train a nurse. Frazier selected Marie Rose, a graduate of the University, as the first nurse anesthetist. Miss Rose, now 90 years old, lives today in

47

Philadelphia and many of the facts quoted have come from her excellent memory. She recalls that Frazier chose her because, "I never cried when scolded and never lost my head when things went wrong." * Miss Rose became the first nurse anesthetist in the State of Pennsylvania (Figure 13).

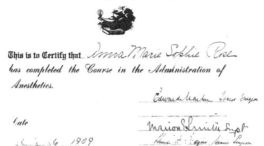

FIGURE. 13. *Photograph of diploma in Anesthetics granted to* MARIE ROSE *in 1909, the first nurse anesthetist in the State of Pennsylvania.*

In 1909, neurosurgeon Frazier wrote [33] :

. . . under no circumstances should an operation be undertaken unless the services of a skilled anesthetizer are available. This problem has been met in my service at the University Hospital by the appointment of a permanent salaried official, a graduate nurse who gives her entire time to the work and has proved eminently satisfactory. In addition to the anesthetizer, the operating room staff includes an assistant, whose duty it is solely to observe and record the blood pressure at frequent intervals throughout the operation.

Resident physicians continued to be pressed into service as anesthetizers if several anesthetics were required simultaneously,[59b] and Edward Beach, a general practitioner, served as a part-time anesthetist for the obstetrical division. Miss Rose taught medical students and remembers among her trainees the eminent professors of medicine Richard Kern, Truman Schnabel, Sr., and Charles Wolferth, all of whom likewise recall her as a competent teacher.

In 1916, Miss Rose's request for an increase in salary was refused,

48

and she left Philadelphia for New York.* Other nurse-anesthetists were then available, since a course of instruction in anesthetics for nurses had begun in 1913.[59c] Until that time, instruction presumably had been individualized. The details of this course are not available. Correspondence from one of the nurses reveals that her instructor in 1920 was I. S. Ravdin.[38] Another note, in 1925, records that the fee for the three-month course was raised from $75 to $100, in order to pay the instructor.[59d]

Not everyone shared White's and Frazier's enthusiasm for nurses as anesthetists, for, in 1912, a Philadelphia medical audience heard Lawrence Irwell, from Buffalo, New York, present "The Case Against the Nurse Anaesthetist".[49] Nonetheless, in 1923, Deaver wrote: [25] "The nurse anesthetist has become an established feature of nearly all surgical services in the country. In my experience, it has proved perfectly satisfactory"; and in 1928, Frazier complimented his "anaesthetizer," Leta Hitz, in a paper [36] describing the use of colonic anesthesia (mixture of paraldehyde, ether, chloretone, and olive oil) for patients "difficult to anesthetize by inhalation." Earlier, he acclaimed the use of paravertebral block, supplemented with ether or nitrous oxide analgesia, for laminectomy,[35] considering this valuable because of previous operative deaths during laminectomy. Frazier continued all his life in favor of nurse anesthesia, and resisted physicians in this capacity.

* Personal communication, M. Rose.

IX

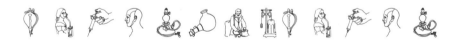

MEN OF VISION

IN 1927, THE SCIENTIFIC LIGHT IN ANESTHESIA AT PENNSYLVANIA WAS rekindled with the appointment of I. S. Ravdin as Director of Surgical

Research. Although accustomed to nurse anesthetists, as well as being one of their instructors and an ardent devotee of spinal anesthesia, Ravdin was keenly aware of some of the fundamental problems of general anesthesia, and set his laboratory to work on them. His encouragement was not confined to his own staff and research laboratories, but he sought and obtained the collaboration of skilled personnel in other disciplines of medicine. In 1926, he, together with internist Richard A. Kern, reported on the "Pulmonary Complications following Anesthesia and Operation." [74] He collaborated with physiologist Samuel Goldschmidt and pathologist Baldwin Lucké in a series of investigations with divinyl ether,[39, 40, 71, 72] and again with the same men in clarifying hepatic toxicity from chloroform.[75, 76] Similarly, he combined with biochemist David Drabkin and obstetrician J. C. Hirst to investigate the effects of barbiturates upon various body organs.[27, 70] Work was also published in concert with pediatricians and pharmacologists on oxygen therapy in relation to phosgene poisoning.[14] Meanwhile, his associates published important papers related to nitrous oxide and hypoxia [73] and experimental spinal anesthesia.[65, 31] The latter paper, by surgeons L. K. Ferguson and J. P. North, was one of the first attempts to place the circulatory changes that follow spinal anesthesia on a physiologic basis. Nearly all these collaborators were to become professors and chairmen of academic departments.

Meanwhile, events were occurring in the Department of Pharmacology that were to have considerable bearing on the future anesthesia department. One of the associates of the renowned pharmacologist, Alfred Newton Richards, was his successor, Carl F. Schmidt, who, with K. K. Chen, first described ephedrine.[28] In the early 1920's, Schmidt envisioned a future in anesthesia and solicited Richards' support. Ravdin was likewise sympathetic, but the ruling surgeons, Frazier and Eliason, were not.* Frustrated with his clinical designs, Schmidt turned his interests to the action of drugs and anesthetics on respiration.[85, 86] He became an authority on the physiology and pharmacology of respiration and of the cerebral circulation. He frequently spoke to and wrote for audiences of anesthetists.[82-84] He did not have an opportunity again to further his own discarded goal in anesthesia, but, in 1938, Richards' laboratory became the environment from which the Anesthesia Department has grown. Among the Pharmacology staff at that time were Julius Comroe, Robert Dripps and Paul Dumke. These three, with Schmidt, worked closely together, establishing a bond of friendship and collaborative effort that continues. As Dripps and Dumke moved into anesthesia, Seymour Kety, James Eckenhoff, Christian Lambertsen, Merel Harmel, George Koelle and Charles Landmesser were to join with Schmidt and Comroe for varying periods. Perhaps these relationships explain the direction that interests within the Department of Anesthesia were to take in future years.

* Personal communication, C. F. Schmidt.

X

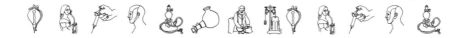

THE FIRST ANESTHESIOLOGIST

LIKEWISE IN 1938, THE FIRST ANESTHESIOLOGIST AT THE UNIVERSITY OF Pennsylvania was appointed. By then, nurses had administered most of the inhalational anesthetics for the previous 30 years. Surgeons gave all spinal anesthetics, while nurses observed the patients during operation, and the Bronchology Department inserted all tracheal tubes. Through Ravdin's insistence, an attempt was made by Professor of Surgery E. L. Eliason to establish a Section of Anesthesiology. Most of the correspondence related to this appears to have been lost, but Milton C. Peterson, then a resident at Bellevue Hospital, was reached in May, 1937, and his interest in coming to Pennsylvania queried.* He was interested and available, but apparently the Board of Managers had not yet approved the idea. In January, 1938, the Medical Board finally appointed a committee to organize a Division of Anesthesiology within the Department of Surgery, the

Section to be in charge of a physician qualified by training in basic sciences which enable him to administer all the modern anesthetics, teach the medi-

51

cal students and internes, and conduct clinical and experimental research in the general subject of gas therapy and anesthesiology.

The Board of Managers approved the request "with the proviso that this department can be operated with a balanced budget." [59e] The concern of the Managers about financing this operation was evident because in March, April and May, there are records of a controversy between that body and the Medical Board concerning anesthetic fees. The physicians refused to set a fee schedule, saying that this was a matter for discussion between patients and their doctors. This probably accounted for the delay in appointing an anesthesiologist, since in March, Eliason, the Professor of Surgery, had written to Peterson informing him that the Trustees had not yet approved the plan, so Peterson withdrew.* The appointment finally went to Ivan B. Taylor, also at Bellevue, who arrived in September, 1938, with the title of Instructor in Surgery and Surgical Assistant at the University Hospital (Figure 14). He was paid a salary of

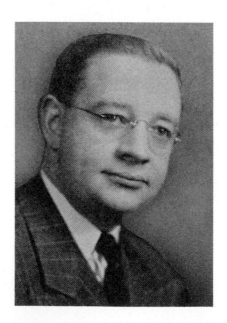

FIGURE 14. IVAN B. TAYLOR, *first anesthesiologist at the University of Pennsylvania, 1938.* (Picture reproduced from the 1941 *Scope.*)

52

$3,500 yearly, and worked full time without private fees.†,[59f] At that time, two diplomates of the American Board of Anesthesiology were in Philadelphia (Ruth and Tyler), and only one other in the State (H. D. Lapp, Reading). Taylor's duties were specifically outlined: † He was to be responsible to the Professor of Surgery and to Hospital Management for the organization and conduct of a department of anesthesiology. He was to examine the patient only at the request of the operating surgeon. He was to confer with the operating surgeon beforehand as to the choice of anesthesia, and was to be responsible to the surgeon during the anesthesia. He was also in charge of gas therapy in the hospital.

Taylor found four nurse anesthetists under the supervision of a head nurse anesthetist, who was responsible to the operating room supervisor and to the surgeon in charge.† The chief nurse anesthetist resigned shortly after Taylor arrived. The surgeons administered spinal anesthesia proficiently, but less skill was demonstrated in caring for the patient during operation. Supplemental general anesthesia was permitted only by the surgeon and usually this was open-drop ether. Teaching was notably lacking. Taylor decided that his main efforts should be to improve clinical anesthesia and to establish a teaching program. At the end of four months, he saw little change in the pattern of anesthesia, but thought that the anesthetics were administered more satisfactorily. He had established an elective course in anesthesia for the medical students, but the attendance was poor and the students refused clinical instruction from nurses. This was overcome by Taylor's doing all the teaching, and by having the students assigned to him personally for two days each in the operating room. This led to criticism from surgeons, that teaching anesthesia in the operating room caused too much confusion. But internes began to apply for two weeks on the anesthesia service.

By the end of a year, Taylor was encouraged by the improvement in clinical anesthesia and in teaching, but was discouraged by his inability to do research or to attract residents. Throughout his second year, things changed but little. The task of one man, responsible for all teaching and clinical supervision, proved frustrating, and his income had not been raised. Simultaneously, late in 1939, the Board of Managers complained that although Taylor was an experienced physician, there had been no increase in anesthesia fees; it thought that fees must be raised so that the hospital could increase Taylor's

53

salary.[59g] Nearly a year later, approval was granted to hire a full-time assistant medical anesthetist provided that a nurse left.[59h] In 1941, Philip Gleason was appointed to the new position, but by this time Taylor had decided to move to Wayne University, giving as reasons for leaving Pennsylvania frustration, inability to get tenure, and Midwestern interests.†

* Personal communication, Milton C. Peterson.
† Personal communication, Ivan B. Taylor.

XI

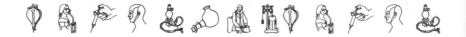

THE CURRENT DEPARTMENT FORMS

THE FUTURE OF ANESTHESIA AT PENNSYLVANIA WAS BEING NURTURED in the Pharmacology Laboratories, separated from this maelstrom. The center of this activity was Robert D. Dripps, who was graduated from Pennsylvania in 1936 and, after a two-year internship at the University Hospital, was appointed Instructor in Pharmacology. At that time, Dripps had no idea of anesthesia as a career, but it was common practice at Pennsylvania to obtain a year or two of background in pharmacology and physiology before returning to clinical practice in medicine. This system, promulgated by Richards, was carried on by Schmidt and is still continued by Koelle and Lambertsen. Innumerable professors of clinical medical specialties throughout the country can point to training by this department. After a year, Dripps was undecided between a career in Pharmacology or in clinical investigation in the Department of Medicine. No stimulation toward anesthesia had come from the hospital, and Taylor had not arrived when

54

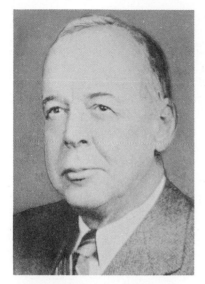

ALFRED NEWTON RICHARDS

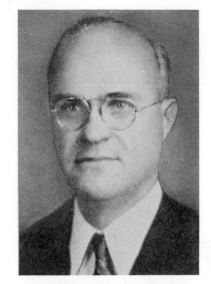

CARL F. SCHMIDT

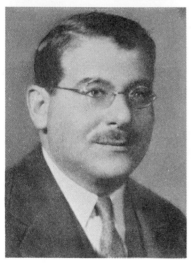

I. S. RAVDIN

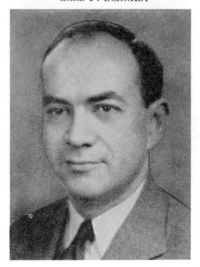

JULIUS H. COMROE

FIGURE 15. *Pictures of* RICHARDS, SCHMIDT *and* COMROE *reproduced from the 1941* Scope, *that of* RAVDIN *from the 1940* Scope.

55

Dripps completed his interneship. However, during the period of indecision, in late 1939, Henry K. Beecher visited the Pharmacology Laboratories.* While informally expounding on the potential in anesthesia, the opportunities for rapid academic advancement, and the relative ease with which a reasonable income could be made, Beecher is alleged to have said: † "I'm scarcely dry behind the ears—and I've written a book, got a Professorship, $8,000 salary and ought to be getting more."

Dripps, ever eager for opportunity, gave quick and decisive thought after this stimulus. He had enjoyed the pharmacology experiments related to anesthesia, and discussions with Schmidt and Ravdin [68] convinced him that opportunity was there. By this time, Richards had become Vice-President in Charge of Medical Affairs, Schmidt was Professor of Pharmacology, and Ravdin was second in command in surgery and seemed heir-apparent. The environment was different from that nearly 20 years earlier, when Schmidt was interested in anesthesiology. Now all three were in positions of authority and, in Dripps, they saw the chance to promote a plan previously agreed on (Figure 15).‡

A Commonwealth Fund Fellowship was obtained for Dripps, and he spent nine months with Ralph Waters at the University of Wisconsin. His future was not yet clearly defined, since he wrote discouragingly to Comroe (Figure 15), who kept the anesthesia fires burning.§ In his long and analytical reply, Comroe dismissed all the alternatives but anesthesia, leaving only the question of clinical practice versus academic anesthesia, with emphasis on research to be considered. He expressed hope that Dripps would return to Philadelphia to do the latter, and offered his full collaboration.†

A few weeks later, the die was cast, and in a report to the Commonwealth Fund, Dripps wrote that he was to return to the Department of Pharmacology to participate in teaching for three months, and then to divide his time between the hospital, as a clinical anesthetist, and the laboratory.§ Further, he projected that his future activities would be in one of three directions: 1. developing research activities in anesthesia as part of the program in anesthesia directed by Taylor; 2. developing a research department of anesthesia under the supervision of the Pharmacology Department; or 3. transferring his clinical activities to the Pennsylvania or Graduate Hospitals and continuing laboratory work at the Medical School.§

Dripps returned to Philadelphia in March, 1941, taught in the Pharmacology course, and continued clinical training as a resident on Taylor's staff. However, with Taylor's resignation, Gleason, who was further advanced in his training than Dripps, was appointed senior anesthetist. The minutes of the Hospital Board read: "Dr. Gleason will by staying until next spring or summer and is senior anesthetist".[59i] This proved prophetic, for shortly after the declaration of War in December, Gleason left the University as anesthetist to the 20th General Hospital Unit without intent of returning, and Dripps was appointed Director of the Department in May, 1942.[59j] At that time, there were still four nurse anesthetists. Margery Van N. Deming came as the first resident in October, 1942.

Life during the war was not easy for the director of this embryonic department. As with Taylor, there was inadequate help, and the attitude of the surgical staff was one of tolerance but hardly encouragement. Ravdin, the principal support among the surgeons, was in India, commanding the 20th General Hospital, clinical responsibilities were heavy, and Dripps's urge to do research was fulfilled during nights and weekends only. Judging from correspondence during the summer of 1945 between Dripps § and Austin Lamont,‖ then Director of Anesthesia at Johns Hopkins University, Dripps, despondent, had just about made up his mind to resign from anesthesia. But Lamont was persuasive, common sense prevailed, and Dripps wrote to Lamont:

. . . in short, I'd better stick to my knitting, keep my trap shut and try to make something of a neglected field. Maybe the two of us could alternately kick each other and keep up the stimulus 'til the war gets over. If things don't improve after the war, we'll be too old to change. I'll become a philosopher, then, and start writing books.

* Personal communication, Henry K. Beecher.
† Personal communication, Julius H. Comroe.
‡ Personal communication, Carl F. Schmidt.
§ Personal communication, Robert D. Dripps.
‖ Personal communication, Austin Lamont.

XII

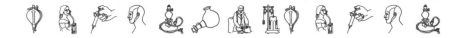

THE WAR'S AFTERMATH

THE NEXT ADDITION TO THE DEPARTMENT WAS JAMES E. ECKENHOFF, WHO, like Dripps, arrived at Pennsylvania influenced by Comroe. Eckenhoff served in the army as an anesthetist with the 107th Evacuation Hospital. In early 1945, while in Germany, he decided on anesthesia as a career, and by chance wrote to Comroe of his decision. Comroe's interest and faith in Dripps's potential is evident from his reply,* as the accuracy of his prophecy is:

I should like to recommend that you consider very strongly coming to the University of Pennsylvania for postgraduate training in anesthesia for a number of reasons. One is that with the close of the war there will be a University Department of Anesthesia on a level with other University departments, a distinction which has been given to very few anesthesia services in the country. As you no doubt know, anesthetists in most hospitals and medical schools are considered as technicians. In the second place, I believe we will have a research organization in anesthesia which will be second to none in the country. This is due to a rather fortunate set of circumstances, for Dr. Schmidt in Pharmacology and Dr. Ravdin in Surgical Research are both interested in backing anesthesia research to the limit. As a result there will be fellowships for two or three years which will consist of fundamental pharmacologic training in research and teaching in Pharmacology with Dr. Schmidt, clinical research in Surgical Research with Dr. Starr, Dripps and me at the University Hospital, and clinical training at the University and Graduate Hospitals. I think that a man will be able to leave our outfit with a better understanding of the problems connected with Anesthesiology (respiratory, circulatory, physiological, etc.) than he would get at any other institution now existing in the country. At any rate think it over and let me know sometime how you feel about it. We are anxious to attract into the field of anesthesia the type of men who can eventually be heads of departments at other medical schools rather than people who are merely disappointed practitioners who have entered anesthesia to make a living.

58

Eckenhoff applied to Comroe for one of the fellowships, and subsequently began his tenure as Harrison Fellow in Anesthesia in November, 1945. He was the first and last such appointment, working in this capacity for one and a half years in the Department of Pharmacology before beginning clinical duties at the University Hospital. He was appointed Assistant Director of the department in 1953, and Professor of Anesthesia in 1955, continuing in these capacities until the end of 1965, when he assumed the Chairmanship of a new Department of Anesthesia at Northwestern University.

As the war ended and physicians returned to civilian life, the anesthetic program began to take shape. In 1946, 12 residents were appointed including Paul Dumke, returned from the Army Chemical Warfare Center. Dumke had served seven years in Pharmacology at Pennsylvania, and was to remain with the anesthesia department until 1953, when he was appointed Director of Anesthesia at Henry Ford Hospital. Charles Landmesser, now Professor of Anesthesia at Albany, also was appointed to the resident staff in 1946. This year saw the organization of a Department of Anesthesia at Children's Hospital in Philadelphia, under Margery Deming. With the influx of physicans to be trained in anesthesia, nurse anesthetists ceased to be part of the clinical program at the University of Pennsylvania.

Some events at the Johns Hopkins Hospital in 1946 also helped to shape destiny at Pennsylvania. Lamont, a graduate of the Hopkins, trained in anesthesia at the University of Wisconsin and with Rovenstine at Bellevue Hospital, was Chief of Anesthesia at the Hopkins from 1943 to 1946. There he had developed a modest program in anesthesia with a parallel nurse-anesthetist's program. He became convinced of the lack of wisdom in training nurses and physicians simultaneously in a university hospital. He prepared a series of proposals to provide Johns Hopkins with a good academic program in anesthesia. Surgeon Blalock refused to agree to the proposals.† Lamont resigned and, in the spring of 1947, accepted the invitation of Dripps to come to Philadelphia. A competent clinician, a widely read scholar, and a person of infinite wisdom, his influence on the Department has been great, although apparent to but few.

Lamont was responsible for bringing two others to Pennsylvania. One was Merel Harmel, who had served as an assistant to Lamont.

59

He came in 1946 and remained with Dripps until 1948, when he left to assume the Professorship at Albany Medical College. The other was Leroy Vandam, who, after four years' training in surgery, had spent two years working in circulatory physiology with Richard Bing at Johns Hopkins. Lamont "converted" Vandam to anesthesia. He came to Pennsylvania as a resident in 1947 and continued on the staff until 1954, when he was appointed Director of Anaesthesia at the Peter Bent Brigham Hospital, Boston, and later Clinical Professor of Anaesthesia at Harvard University.

At the time of Ivan Taylor's appointment at Pennsylvania, Frederick Haugen became Chief of Anesthesiology at the Presbyterian Hospital in Philadelphia. He remained in this position until 1948, when he accepted the Professorship at the University of Oregon. Among his residents were H. H. Stone, Benton D. King, and H. L. Price. Stone was a resident during 1943 and 1944, and on his return from army service, in 1946, was appointed Director of Anesthesia at the University of Pennsylvania Graduate Hospital. He was the third physician to have charge of that unit.‡ The first, Edward Beach, a general practitioner and part-time anesthetist, had worked before 1925 at the University Hospital. That year he moved his interests to the Graduate Hospital and established an eight-months course for nurse anesthetists. In 1935, he confined his practice to anesthesia until he died, in 1944. Dripps acted as nominal chief of the service after this until Stone's appointment, although he gave few anesthetics there.

King was a resident with Haugen during 1945-1946, and came to Pennsylvania in 1946, where he was to remain until 1952. After two years' service in the army, he was appointed Professor at the State University of New York at Buffalo. Price was a resident during 1947-1948, when Haugen decided to move to Oregon. He had not finished his training when he was called into the Army. After two years of service, he returned to Pennsylvania, completed his training, was appointed a Research Associate and, shortly thereafter, awarded a National Research Council Fellowship in Physiology at Harvard University. On his return a year later, he was appointed Assistant Professor of Anesthesiology and since then has devoted nearly full time

60

to research in the specialty. In 1961, he was made Professor of Anesthesia.

* Personal communication, Julius H. Comroe.
† Personal communication, Austin Lamont.
‡ Personal communication, H. H. Stone.

XIII

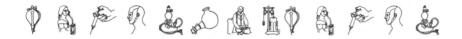

A GENERATION WITH DRIPPS

The current Department of Anesthesia has continued the scientific approach to anesthesia that has prevailed since the days of James

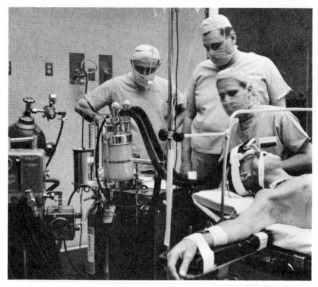

FIGURE 16. *Practical instruction in the administration of anesthetics at the Hospital of the University of Pennsylvania, 1965.*

61

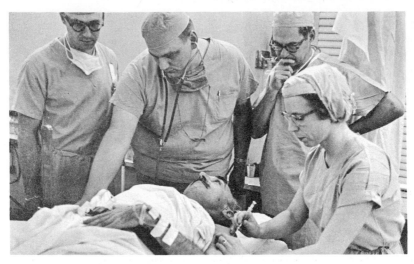

FIGURE 17. *Clinical investigation on the effect of narcotic analgesics in the Recovery Room of the Hospital of the University of Pennsylvania.*

Woodhouse. The literature on anesthetics that has originated at Pennsylvania relates, in the main, to the physiology and pharmacology of anesthesia; clinical articles appear, but are in the minority.[122] A healthy skepticism has dominated the Pennsylvania faculty since the introduction of surgical anesthesia. The emphasis has always been on teaching fundamentals and on encouraging students to think clearly, observe carefully, and make measurements (Figures 16-23). Perhaps this same spirit was inculcated in Crawford Long and explains his reticence to report his experiences.

Since the days of Horatio Wood, Jr., close relationships have been maintained with the Departments of Pharmacology and Medicine. Until Ravdin's tenure, the surgeons contributed little to the growth of anesthesia and perhaps retarded it significantly. Yet it was Ravdin, a man of vision,[68, 69] together with the eminent physiologically minded pharmacologists, Richards and Schmidt, who recognized the need for a properly oriented physician to head a Department of Anesthesia. As these three men look back on the organization that has grown from their imaginations, they must feel pleasure and pride.

Since 1945, 280 residents or fellows have been trained. Whereas at the end of World War II only two physicians were in the Depart-

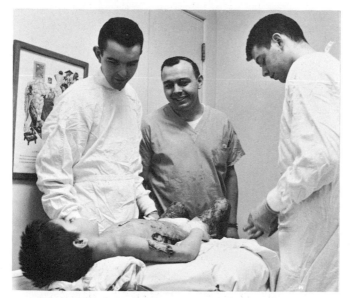

FIGURE 18. *Participation in Total Patient Care. Great emphasis has always been laid on the principle that the anesthetist is a physician with responsibilities outside as well as within the operating room.*

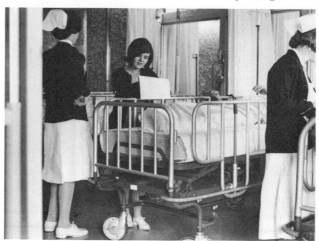

FIGURE 19. *The Postanesthetic Recovery Room at the Hospital of the University of Pennsylvania under the direction of the Department of Anesthesia.*

63

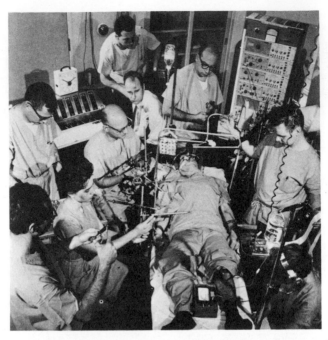

FIGURE 20. *Investigation on cerebal circulation and cerebral metabolism by members of the Department of Anesthesia under the direction of* DR. HARRY WOLLMAN.

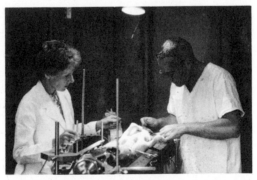

FIGURE 21. *Experiment in fundamental anesthetic research by* PROFESSOR HENRY L. PRICE *and Research Associate* MARY L. PRICE. *The department maintains its own animal research laboratories, where Dr. Price has conducted his research related to catecholamines and the effect of anesthetic agents on the circulation.*

64

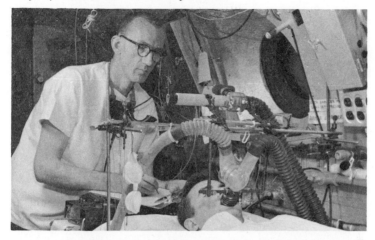

FIGURE 22. *Experiment in hyperbaric medicine by* DR. JAMES DICKSON, *formerly a member of the Department of Anesthesia. These investigations are conducted in the Pharmacology Department, under the direction of* PROFESSOR CHRISTIAN J. LAMBERTSEN, *with residents and staff of the Anesthesia Department participating.*

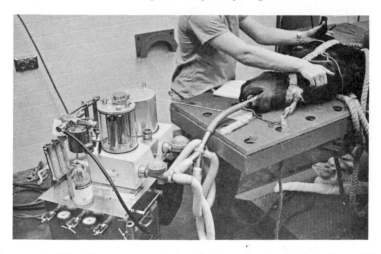

FIGURE 23. *The Department of Anesthesia at Pennsylvania points with pride to having trained the first veterinarian anesthesiologist in the United States,* DR. LAWRENCE R. SOMA. *An anesthetic is pictured above in progress at the New Bolton Center, University of Pennsylvania. Dr. Soma's department at the Veterinary School maintains close laison with the University's Anesthesia Department.*

ment, now it has 15 staff anesthesiologists, 34 residents and fellows, and two PhD biochemists. Of its former members, 74 hold academic positions in American and foreign medical schools, 13 of them as departmental chairmen. From the Department's laboratories and clinics have come 309 publications (see *Bibliography 1943–1965*). Its staff members and alumni have held and continue to hold prominent positions in local, state and national medical organizations. Five of the staff and alumni serve on National Institutes of Health Advisory Committees, one is consultant to the Surgeon General of the Army, another to the Surgeon General of the Navy, and a third chairman of the National Research Council's Subcommittee on Anesthesia. Two of the alumni have served as editor of *Anesthesiology*, and two are Directors of the American Board of Anesthesiology. The textbook written by Dripps, Eckenhoff and Vandam has proved popular among residents and students, and has sold nearly 26,000 copies in two editions. Finally, the department is recognized as providing one of the outstanding courses of instruction in the University's Medical School.

The possibility of endowment of a professorial chair in anesthesia had been envisaged for years, and finally came into reality at the end of 1965. Robert Lincoln McNeil (portrait opposite), a graduate of the University of Pennsylvania in 1904, is former president of McNeil Laboratories, Inc. Mr. McNeil is one of two men to have served as president of both the American Pharmaceutical Manufacturers Association and the American Drug Manufacturers Association. He was joined by Mrs. McNeil, the former Grace F. Slack, of Bethel, Connecticut, in the establishment of the chair. Their friendship with Dr. Dripps has been lifelong, beginning in 1918 when Mr. McNeil taught Dripps in the Sunday School of the First Presbyterian Church of Germantown. The two families have been close to one another through three generations, with Dripps acting as professional consultant for almost 25 years and the McNeils offering counsel, guidance, and warm personal interest in return. The chair, created in recognition of the achievement of Dripps and his department, is a natural climax of the deep bond that holds together the McNeil and the Dripps families in mutual respect and affection.

66

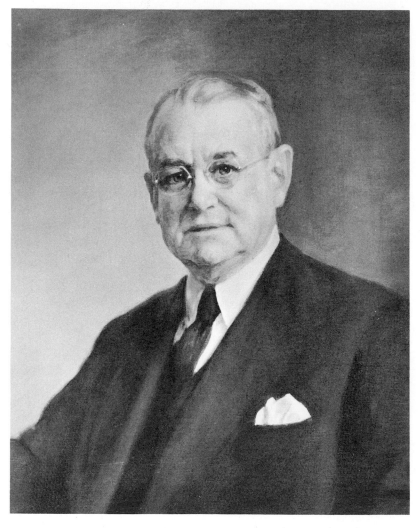

OIL PAINTING BY LAZAR RADITZ

ROBERT LINCOLN McNEIL

XIV

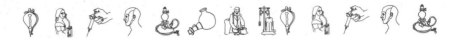

RECAPITULATION

THE CHALLENGES IN THE FORMATION OF THE DEPARTMENT OF ANESTHESIA at Pennsylvania have been similar to those at other universities. The beginning was harassing, with the first director leaving in frustration and his successor doubting the wisdom of specializing in anesthesia. The problem of recruitment of competent men weighed heavily, and there was an uphill battle to establish clinical and research competence as well as professional stature. Nothing came by mandate. Every gain was from painstaking planning and quiet demonstration of excellence in patient care, teaching students, and research and administration. Taylor, lacking in research training, was prepared to upgrade clinical anesthesia but was unwilling to accept the harassment of building a department without encouragement. Dripps was endowed with the ability to teach and trained to do research. The four years he served with minimal professional help gave him an opportunity to gain clinical skill. During this period, he was the author or co-author of 12 publications, eight of which dealt with fundamentals of anesthesia. This work was mostly with the help of Julius Comroe, who promised his support and kept his word. Dripps was fortunate that the war ended when it did, providing a pool of residents for training in anesthesia. He was farsighted enough to send some of these individuals into the laboratory, despite his urgent need for clinical assistance. He was helped, too, by the coincidence of Lamont's leaving the Hopkins and Haugen's moving to Oregon. His firm belief that anesthesiology was essentially clinical pharmacology and physiology, and that men trained in these basic disciplines would make better anesthetists, teachers, and investigators, has proved wise and fruitful. He has built one of the truly great departments of anesthesia in the world.

68

XV

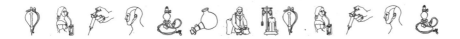

BIBLIOGRAPHY

1. Adams, J. H.: Life of D. Hayes Agnew. Philadelphia, F. A. Davis Co., 1892.

2. Agnew, D. H.: Principles and Practice of Surgery. Philadelphia, J. B. Lippincott Co., 1881, Vol. 2, pp. 280-292.

3. Artusio, J. F.: Di-ethyl ether analgesia: A detailed description of the first stage of ether anesthesia in man, J Pharmacol Exp Ther *111*:343, 1954.

4. Ashhurst, J.: Principles and Practice of Surgery. Philadelphia, Lea Bros., 6th ed., 1893, pp. 83-92.

5. Ashhurst, J., Jr.: Surgery before the days of anaesthesia, Int Med Mag *5*: 545, 1896.

6. Babcock, W. W.: Spinal anesthesia—clinical study of 658 administrations, Penn Med J *12*:891, 1909.

7. ———: Dangers and disadvantages of spinal anesthesia, New York J Med *98*:897, 1913.

8. Barton, W. P. C.: A Dissertation on the Chymical Properties and Exhilarating Effects of Nitrous Oxide Gas: and Its Application to Pneumatick Medicine. Philadelphia, Lorenzo Press, 1808.

9. Bibliographical notices, Art. XVII, Am J Med Sci *30*:486, 1848.

10. Bibliographical notices, Art, XVIII, Am J Med Sci *30*:493, 1848.

11. Blochman, L. G.: Doctor Squibb. The Life and Times of a Rugged Idealist. New York, Simon and Schuster, 1958.

12. Boland, F. K.: The First Anaesthetic. Athens (Georgia) University of Georgia Press, 1950.

13. Bolton, H. C.: Scientific Correspondence of Joseph Priestley. Privately printed, New York, 1892, p. 144.

14. Bruner, H. D., Boche, R. D., Chapple, C. C., Gibbon, M. H., and McCarthy, M. D.: Studies on experimental phosgene poisoning, J Clin Invest *26*: 936, 1947.

15. Burr, A. R.: Weir Mitchell, His Life and Letters. New York, Duffield & Co., 1929, p. 45.

16. Carpenter, J. T.: Chloroform anaesthesia, Univ Med Mag *2*:457, 1890.

17. Carson, J.: A History of the Medical Department of the University of Pennsylvania. Philadelphia, Lindsay & Blakiston, 1869.

18. Catalogue of the Alumni of the Medical Department of the University of Pennsylvania. Philadelphia, Collins, Printer, 1877.

19. Chapman, N.: Elements of Therapeutics and Materia Medica. Philadelphia, Carey & Lea, 1831.

20. Chen, K. K., and Schmidt, C. F.: The action of ephedrine, the active principle of the Chinese drug, ma huang, J Pharmacol Exp Ther 24:339, 1924.

21. Corner, G. W.: Two Centuries of Medicine. Philadelphia, J. B. Lippincott Co., 1965.

22. Coxe, E. J.: A Practical Treatise on Medical Inhalation. Philadelphia, Thomas Dobson, 1841.

23. Coxe, J. R.: The American Dispensatory. Philadelphia, Thomas Dobson, 2nd ed., 1810.

24. Davy, H.: Researches, Chemical and Physiological; Chiefly Concerning Nitrous Oxide or Dephlogisticated Nitrous Air and Its Respiration. London, Johnson, 1800.

25. Deaver, J. B.: Excursions into Surgical Subjects. Philadelphia, W. B. Saunders Co., 1923, p. 111.

26. Deaver, J. B., and Frese, C.: The influence of ether narcosis upon the genito-urinary tract, Univ Med Mag 7:750, 1894.

27. Drabkin, D. L., Ravdin, I. S., Hirst, J. C., and Lapham, M. E.: The effect of amytal anesthesia upon the uterus and its use in obstetrics, Am J Med Sci 178:379, 1929.

28. Duncum, B. M.: The Development of Inhalational Anaesthesia. New York, Oxford University Press, 1947.

29. Eckenhoff, J. E.: The anesthetists in Thomas Eakins' "Clinics," Anesthesiology 26:663, 1965.

30. Ether inhalation as a means of annulling pain, Am J Med Sci 28:512, 1847.

31. Ferguson, L. K., and North, J. P.: Observations on experimental spinal anaesthesia, Surg Gynec Obstet 54:621, 1932.

32. Foreign Correspondence: Am J Med Sci 27:500, 1847.

33. Frazier, C. H.: Problems and procedures in cranial surgery, JAMA 52:1805, 1909.

34. ———: Resuscitation by cardiac massage, JAMA 56:1448, 1911.

35. ———: Laminectomy and regional anaesthesia, Ann Surg 68:12, 1918.

36. ———: Colonic anaesthesia in operations upon brain and spinal cord, Ann Surg 87:161, 1928.

37. Gillespie, J.: Does ether kill? Phila Med Times 11:772, 1881.

38. Goff, A. C.: Personal communication.

39. Goldschmidt, S., Ravdin, I. S., and Lucke, B.: Anesthesia, and liver damage. I. The protective action of oxygen against the necrotizing effect of certain anesthetics on the liver, J Pharmacol Exp Ther 59:1, 1937.

40. Goldschmidt, S., Ravdin, I. S., Lucke, B., Muller, G. O., Johnston, C. G., and Ruigh, W. L.: Divinyl ether, JAMA 102:21, 1934.

41. Hamblen, R. N.: The occurrence of acetonuria following ether anesthesia, Univ Pennsylvania Med Bull 22:147, 1909.

42. Hare, H. A.: The cause of the arrest of respiration in the early stages of ether anesthesia, Univ Med Mag 1:419, 1888.

43. ———: Experiments to determine the influence of etherization on the normal bodily temperature with reference to the use of external heat, Ther Gaz 12:317, 1888.

44. Hare, R.: A Compendium of the Course of Chemical Instruction in the Medical Department of the University of Pennsylvania. Philadelphia, J. G. Auner, 1836, pp. 226-227.

45. Hartshorne, E.: Remarks on the case of a dentist convicted of violating a patient while under influence of ether inhalation, Med Examiner *10* (N.S.): 705, 1854.

46. Hartshorne, H.: Notes on hospital practice, Am J Med. Sci *16*:353, 1848.

47. ———: Influence of ether on the nervous centers, Tr Coll Phys Phila *2*: 331, 1854.

48. Hodge, H. L.: Principles and Practice of Obstetrics. Philadelphia, Blanchard & Lea, 1864, p. 429.

49. Irwell, L.: The case against the nurse anesthetist, Int Clin *2*:(22 series)157, 1912.

50. Kean, W. W.: Address to Medical and Chirurgical Faculty of State of Maryland, April, 1899.

51. Krumbhaar, E. B.: Medical Student Notes, 1908, on file in Library of College of Physicians, Philadelphia.

52. Littell, S.: George Bacon Wood, Tr Coll Phys Phila *5*:(3rd series)25, 1881.

53. Ludovici, L. J.: The Discovery of Anaesthesia. New York, Thomas Y. Crowell Co., 1961.

54. Lyman, H. M.: Anaesthetics and Anaesthesia, *in* International Encyclopedia of Surgery, edited by J. Ashhurst, New York, William Wood and Co., vol. 1, 1881.

55. ———: Artificial Anaesthesia and Anaesthetics. New York, William Wood, 1881.

56. Martin, E., and Hare, H. A.: The treatment of arrested respiration in anaesthesia, Med News *54*:236, 1889.

57. Medical Record *51*:574, 1897.

58. Memorial to Dr. Crawford W. Long: Univ Pennsylvania Med Bull(12th series)No. 4, Part 9, 1912.

59. Minutes of Executive Committee of Board of Managers, Hospital of the University of Pennsylvania: a) Dec 17, 1908; b) Dec 11, 1909; c) June 5, 1913; d) April 16, 1925; e) Jan 19, 1938; f) Sept 21, 1938; g) July 19, 1939; h) Dec 18, 1940; i) Sept 17, 1941; j) May 20, 1942.

60. Mitchell, S. W.: On a rare vaso-motor neurosis of the extremities, and on the maladies with which it may be confounded, Am J Med Sci *76*:17, 1878.

61. ———: The Birth and Death of Pain. Anaesthesia Semi-Centennial. Cambridge (Mass), H. O. Houghton & Co., 1897.

62. Mitchell, S. W., Keen, W. W., and Morehouse, G. R.: On the Antagonism of atropia and morphia, Am J Med Sci *50*:67, 1865.

63. Norris, C. C.: Preliminary anaesthesia by nitrous oxide gas. Report of 150 cases by this method compared with 150 cases of plain etherization, Univ Pennsylvania Med Bull *15*:178, 1902.

64. Norris, H.: Scopolamine-morphine anaesthesia, Univ Pennsylvania Med Bull *18*:234, 1905.

65. North, J. P.: Use and abuse of spinal anesthesia, Ann Surg *101*:702, 1935.

66. Packard, F. R.: The Conquest of Surgical Pain. Lancaster (Pa), Lancaster Press, 1940.

67. Pleadwell, F. L.: William Paul Crillion Barton, Surgeon, US Navy, a pioneer in American Naval Medicine, Ann Med Hist *2*:267, 1919.

68. Ravdin, I. S.: Editorial: A surgeon comments on the specialty of anesthesiology, Anesthesiology *2*:207, 1941.

69. ————: Editorial: Anesthesiologists, surgeons and malpractice suits, Anesthesiology *20*:377, 1959.

70. Ravdin, I. S., Drabkin, D. L., and Bothe, A. E.: The effect of repeated injections of sodium iso-amyl-ethyl barbiturate on various viscera, J Lab Clin Med *16*:561, 1931.

71. Ravdin, I. S., Eliason, E. L., Coates, G. M., Halloway, T. B., Ferguson, L. K., Gill, A. B., and Cook, T. J.: Divinyl ether—a report of its further use as a general anesthetic, JAMA *108*:1163, 1937.

72. ———— Further experience with vinethene anesthesia, Anesth Analg (Cleveland) *17*:176, 1938.

73. Ravdin, I. S., and Johnston, C. G.: Nitrous oxide—oxygen anesthesia and anoxia, Am J Med Sci *194*:279, 1937.

74. Ravdin, I. S., and Kern, R. A.: Pulmonary complications following anesthesia and operation: A statistical study, Arch Surg (Chicago) *13*:120, 1926

75. Ravdin, I. S., Vars, H. M., and Goldschmidt, S.: The non-specificity of suspension of sodium xanthine in protecting the liver against injury by chloroform, and the probable course of its action, J Clin Invest *18*:633, 1939.

76. Ravdin, I. S., Vars, H. M., Goldschmidt, S., and Klingensmith, L. E.: Anesthesia and liver damage. II. The effect of anesthesia on the blood sugar, the liver glycogen and liver fat, J Pharmacol Exp Ther *64*:111, 1938.

77. Roberts, J. B.: Ether deaths: A personal experience in four cases of death from anaesthetics, Phila Med Times *11*:545, 1881.

78. ————: The anesthesia peril in American hospitals, Ther Gaz *32*:89, 1908.

79. Rush, B.: Lectures on Medicine, 2 vols., Philadelphia, undated. Title page missing. On file at Library of College of Physicians, Philadelphia.

80. ————: Six Introductory Lectures to Course of Lectures upon the Institutes and Practice of Medicine. Philadelphia, John Conrad & Co., 1801.

81. ————: Syllabus of a Course of Lectures upon Physiology, Pathology, Therapeutics and the Practice of Medicine. Philadelphia, John Conrad & Co., 1801.

82. Schmidt, C. F.: Recent studies on some physiological phenomena related to anesthesia, Anesth Analg (Cleveland) *17*:2, 1938.

83. ————: The revolution in respiratory physiology, Anesthesiology *5*:77, 1944.

84. ————: Recent developments in respiratory physiology related to anesthesia, Anesthesiology *6*:113, 1945.

85. Schmidt, C. F., and Harer, W. B.: The action of drugs on respiration. I. The morphine series, J Exp Med *37*:47, 1923.

86. ————: The action of drugs on respiration. II. Ether, chloroform, chloral, urethane, luminal, magnesium, caffeine, strychnine, and atropine, J Exp Med *37*: 69, 1923.

87. Silliman, B.: Elements of Chemistry. New Haven, H. Howe, 1830.

88. Smith, D. F.: James Woodhouse, a Pioneer in Chemistry. Philadelphia, John C. Winston, 1918.

89. Smith, H. H.: System of Operative Surgery. Philadelphia, Lippincott, Grambo & Co., 1st ed., 1852.

90. ————. Principles and Practice of Surgery. Philadelphia, J. B. Lippincott Co., 1863.

91. Stillé, A.: Therapeutics and Materia Medica. Philadelphia, H. C. Lea, 4th ed., 1874, pp. 77–164.

92. Stillé, M.: The psychical effects of ether inhalation, Med Examiner *10:* (N.S.)730, 1854.

93. Stockton, E. B.: Essence of Dr. Rush's Lectures, Winter, 1815–16, Philadelphia, 1817. Notebook on file at Library of College of Physicians, Philadelphia.

94. Symposium on Anaesthetics, Int Clin *2:*(22 series)157, 1912.

95. Taylor, F. L.: Crawford W. Long and the Discovery of Ether Anaesthesia. New York, Paul Hoeber, 1928.

96. Testimonial of Members of the Medical Profession of Philadelphia in Behalf of Wm. T. G. Morton, Feb 15, 1860. Philadelphia, Collins, 1860.

97. The Lancet and the Hyderabad Commission on Chloroform. London, Lancet, 1895.

98. Warren, J. C.: Inhalation of ethereal vapour for the prevention of pain in surgical operations, Am J Med Sci 27:260, 1847.

99. White, J. W.: Anaesthetics, Med & Surg Reporter *60:*289, 1889.

100. Wood, G. B.: Syllabus on Course of Lectures on Materia Medica and Pharmacy. Philadelphia, Bailey, 1847.

101. ———: A Treatise on Therapeutics and Pharmacology or Materia Medica. Philadelphia, J. B. Lippincott Co., 1856.

102. Wood, G. B., and Bache, F.: United States Dispensatory. Philadelphia, Grigg and Eliott, vol. 2, 4th ed., 1839.

103. Wood, G. B., Jr.: The elimination of ether and its relation to the kidney, Univ Med Mag *6:*802, 1893.

104. Wood, H. C.: Acetic ether as an anaesthetic, Am J Med Sci *60:*137, 1870.

105. ———: Clinical lecture on the treatment of opium poisoning. Phila Med Times *6:*145, 1875.

106. ———. Therapeutics, Its Principles and Practice. Philadelphia, J. B. Lippincott Co., 1875.

107. ———: Therapeutics: Its Principles and Practice. Philadelphia, J. B. Lippincott Co., 7th ed., 1888.

108. ———: Anaesthesia—paper before the 10th International Medical Congress, Berlin, Med News *57:*121, 1890.

109. ———: Anaesthesia, Anesthesia *7:*1, 1891.

110. ———: Chloroform anesthesia, Tr Coll Phys Phila *15:*198, 1893.

111. ———: On the action of nitrous oxide and of the mixture of nitrous oxide and oxygen, Dental Cosmos *35:*1, 1893.

112. ———: Anaesthesia, in System of Surgery, edited by F. S. Dennis, Philadelphia, Lea Bros & Co., vol. 1, 1895, p. 645.

113. ———: Benzine in anaesthetic mixtures, Phila Med J *3:*843, 1899.

114. Wood, H. C., and Carter, W. S.: A research upon anaesthesia, J Exp Med *2:*131, 1897.

115. Wood, H. C., and Cerna, D.: Chloride of ethyl and pental, Phila Co Med Soc Proc *13:*1, 1892.

116. ———: The effects of drugs and other agencies upon the respiratory movements, J Physiol (London) (Paris) *13:*870, 1892.

117. Wood, H. C., and Hare, H. A.: The cause of death from chloroform, Med News *56:*190, 1890.

118. Wood, H. C., and Hoyt, D. M.: The action of alcohol upon the circulation, Univ Pennsylvania Med Bull *18:*70, 1905.

119. Wood, H. C., Jr.: Contribution to our knowledge of the physiological action of atropia, Amer J Med Sci *65:*332, 1873.

120. ——: A study of the effect of minute doses of ether and chloroform, Univ Med Mag *10:595*, 1897.

121. Woodward, G. S.: The Man Who Conquered Pain. Boston, Beacon Press, 1962.

122. Eckenhoff, J. E., ed.: Science and Practice in Anesthesia. Philadelphia, J. B. Lippincott Co., 1965.

123. Transactions of the Amer Med Ass *1:215–219*, 1848.

Bibliography

Department of Anesthesia University of Pennsylvania 1943 to 1965

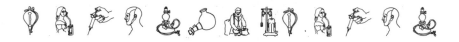

1. Dripps, R. D. and Dumke, P. R.: The effect of narcotics on the balance between central and chemoreceptor control of respiration, J Pharmacol Exp Ther 77:290, 1943.

2. Dripps, R. D.: The pharmacological basis for preoperative medication, Surg Clin N Am, 1377, 1944.

3. Comroe, J. H., Jr. and Dripps, R. D.: The oxygen tension of arterial blood and alveolar air in normal human subjects, Am J Physiol *142*:700, 1944.

4. Dripps, R. D. and Comroe, J. H., Jr.: The clinical significance of the carotid and aortic bodies, Am J Med Sci *208*:681, 1944.

5. Dripps, R. D.: How can I "keep up" with medical progress, Anesthesiology 6:81, 1945.

6. Dripps, R. D. and Comroe, J. H., Jr.: Clinical studies on morphine. I. The immediate effect of morphine administered intravenously and intramuscularly upon the respiration of normal man, Anesthesiology, 6:462, 1945.

7. Comroe, J. H., Jr. and Dripps, R. D.: Applied physiology, Ann Rev Physiol 7:653, 1945.

8. Comroe, J. H., Jr., Dripps, R. D., Dumke, P. R. and Deming, M.: Oxygen toxicity, JAMA *128*:710, 1945.

9. Drew, J. H., Dripps, R. D. and Comroe, J. H., Jr.: Clinical studies on morphine. II. The effect of morphine upon the circulation of man and upon the circulatory and respiratory response to tilting, Anesthesiology 7:44, 1946.

10. Comroe, J. H., Jr. and Dripps, R. D.: Artificial respiration, JAMA *130:*381, 1946.

11. ———: The histamine-like action of curare and tubocurarine injected intracutaneously and intra-arterially in man, Anesthesiology 7:260, 1946.

12. Dripps, R. D. and Deming, M.: Postoperative atelectasis and pneumonia, Ann Surg 124:94, 1946.

13. ———: An evaluation of certain drugs used to maintain blood pressure during spinal anesthesia, Surg Gynec Obstet 83:312, 1946.

14. Dripps, R. D.: Circulatory changes during spinal anesthesia: Their physiological basis, Surg Clin N Am, Dec, 1946.

15. Dripps, R. D. and Comroe, J. H., Jr.: Circulatory physiology—the adjustment to blood loss and postural changes, Surg Clin N Am 1368, 1946.

16. Dripps, R. D.: The immediate decrease of blood pressure seen at the conclusion of cyclopropane anesthesia: "Cyclopropane shock," Anesthesiology 8: 15, 1947.

17. Eckenhoff, J. E., Hafkenschiel, J. H. and Landmesser, C. M.: The coronary circulation in the dog, Am J Physiol 148:582, 1947.

18. Dripps, R. D. and Comroe, J. H., Jr.: The respiratory and circulatory response of normal man to inhalation of 7.6 and 10.4 per cent CO_2 with a comparison of the maximal ventilation produced by severe muscular exercise, inhalation of CO_2 and maximal voluntary hyperventilation, Am J Physiol 149:43, 1947.

19. ———: The effect of the inhalation of high and low oxygen concentrations on respiration, pulse rate, ballistocardiogram and arterial oxygen saturation (oximeter) of normal individuals, Am J Physiol 149:277, 1947.

20. Dripps, R. D. and Sergent, W. F.: Use of a new curarizing agent, dihydrobetaerythroidine for the production of muscular relaxation during anesthesia and surgery, Anesthesiology 8:241, 1947.

21. Eckenhoff, J. E., Hafkenschiel, J. H., Landmesser, C. M. and Harmel, M. H.: Cardiac oxygen metabolism and control of the coronary circulation, Am J Physiol 149:634, 1947.

22. Comroe, J. H., Jr. and Dripps, R. D.: Curare and curare-like compounds, Surg Clin N Am 1575, 1947.

23. Eckenhoff, J. E. and Hafkenschiel, J. H.: The effect of nikethamide on coronary blood flow and cardiac oxygen metabolism, J Pharmacol Exp Ther 91: 362, 1947.

24. Dripps, R. D. and Dumke, P. R.: Recent advances in anesthesia, Surg Clin N Am 1566, 1947.

25. Comroe, J. H., Jr., Dripps, R. D., Botelho, S. and Rubin, H. M.: The curare-like action of ether upon the human neuromuscular transmission, Fed Proc 6:318, 1947.

26. Turville, C. S. and Dripps, R. D.: The anesthetic management of the aged, Penn Med J 51:434, 1948.

27. Eckenhoff, J. E., Hafkenschiel, J. H., Harmel, M. H., Goodale, W. T., Lubin, M., Bing, R. J. and Kety, S. S.: The measurement of coronary blood flow by the nitrous oxide method, Am J Physiol 152:356, 1948.

28. Eckenhoff, J. E., Hafkenschiel, J. H., Foltz, E. L. and Driver, R. L.: The influence of hypotension on coronary blood flow, cardiac work and cardiac efficiency, Am J Physiol 152:545, 1948.

29. Landmesser, C. M. and Dripps, R. D.: A new method for recording the effect of various agents upon the caliber of the human bronchial tree, Anesthesiology 9:159, 1948.

76

30. Dripps, R. D., Kirby, C. K., Johnson, J. and Erb. W. N.: Cardiac resuscitation, Ann Surg *127:*592, 1948.

31. Comroe, J. H., Jr. and Dripps, R. D.: Reactions to morphine in ambulatory and bed patients, Surg Gynec Obstet *87:*221, 1948.

32. Eckenhoff, J. E. and Hafkenschiel, J. H.: The oxygen content of coronary venous blood as affected by anoxia and cytochrome C Am Heart J *36:*893, 1948.

33. Dripps, R. D.: Selective utilization of barbiturates: As illustrated by a study of butabarbital sodium (NNR), JAMA *139:*148, 1949.

34. Dripps, R. D.: Lung function, Am J Roentgen *61:*23, 1949.

35. Kirby, C. K., Eckenhoff, J. E. and Looby, J.: The use of hyaluronidase with local anesthetic agents in nerve block and infiltration anesthesia, Surgery *25:* 101, 1949.

36. Eather, K. F., Peterson, L. H. and Dripps, R. D.: Studies of the circulation of anesthetized patients by a new method for recording arterial pressure and pressure pulse contours, Anesthesiology *10:*125, 1949.

37. Eckenhoff, J. E., Schmidt, C. F., Dripps, R. D. and Kety, S. S.: A status report on analeptics, JAMA *139:*780, 1949.

38. Peterson, L. H., Dripps, R. D. and Risman, G. C.: A method for recording the arterial pressure pulse and blood pressure in man, Am Heart J *37:*771, 1949.

39. Sergeant, W. F. and Dripps, R. D.: Attempts to prolong and intensify spinal anesthesia by the addition of ephedrine, neosynephrine or epinephrine to a pontocaine-glucose solution, Anesthesiology *10:*260, 1949.

40. Dripps, R. D.: Spinal anesthesia for diagnosis and therapy, Veterans Administration Tech Bull, June 13, 1949.

41. Dripps, R. D.: Research and its relationship to clinical anesthesia, Anesthesiology *10:*690, 1949.

42. Dripps, R. D.: Medicine of the Year—Anesthesiology Section, Philadelphia, J. B. Lippincott, 1949.

43. Peterson, L. H., Eather, K. F. and Dripps, R. D.: Postural changes in the circulation of surgical patients as studied by a new method for recording the arterial blood pressure and pressure pulse, Ann Surg *131:*23, 1950.

44. Eckenhoff, J. E.: Physiology of the coronary circulation, Anesthesiology *11:*168, 1950.

45. Dripps, R. D.: Medicine of the Year—Anesthesiology Section, Philadelphia, J. B. Lippincott, 1950.

46. ———: A comparison of the malleable needle and catheter technics for continuous spinal anesthesia, New York J Med *50:*1595, 1950.

47. King, B. D. and Dripps, R. D.: The use of methoxamine for maintenance of the circulation during spinal anesthesia, Surg Gynec Obstet *90:*659, 1950.

48. Harris, L. C., Jr. and Dripps, R. D.: The use of decamethonium bromide for the production of muscular relaxation, Anesthesiology *11:*215, 1950.

49. Conner, E. H. and Dripps, R. D.: The use of lucaine in the study of spinal anesthesia, Anesthesiology *11:*686, 1950.

50. Peterson, L. H.: Some characteristics of the certain reflexes which modify the circulation in man, Circulation *2:*351, 1950.

51. Eckenhoff, J. E. and Kirby, C. K.: The use of hyaluronidase in regional nerve blocks, Anesthesiology *12:*27, 1951.

52. Rubin, A., Winston, J., Metz-Rubin, H. and Berwick, L.: The vestibular response to turning with nomograms for the detection of streptomycin and other drug toxicities and for the prediction of the normal variations of nystagmus and vertigo, Ann Otol 60:108, 1951.

53. Rubin, A. and Metz-Rubin, H.: The effect of dramamine upon postoperative nausea and vomiting, Surg Gynec Obstet 92:415, 1951.

54. Wechsler, R. L., Dripps, R. D. and Kety, S. S.: Blood flow and oxygen consumption of the human brain during anesthesia produced by thiopental, Anesthesiology 12:308, 1951.

55. Johnson, J., Kirby, C. K. and Dripps, R. D.: Defibrillation of the ventricles by electric shock with complete recovery, Ann Surg 134:116, 1951.

56. Eckenhoff, J. E.: Some anatomic considerations of the infant larynx influencing endotracheal anesthesia, Anesthesiology 12:401, 1951.

57. Dripps, R. D. and Vandam, L. D.: Postlumbar puncture headache, Chicago Med Soc Bull, Aug, 1951.

58. King, B. D., Harris, L. C., Jr., Greifenstein, F. E., Elder, J. D., Jr. and Dripps, R. D.: Reflex circulatory response to direct laryngoscopy and tracheal intubation during general anesthesia, Anesthesiology 12:556, 1951.

59. Dripps, R. D. and Vandam, L. D.: Hazards of lumbar puncture, JAMA 147:1118, 1951.

60. Price, H. L., King, B. D., Elder, J. D., Jr., Libien, B. H. and Dripps, R. D.: Circulatory effects of raised airway pressure during cyclopropane anesthesia in man, J Clin Invest 30:1243, 1951.

61. Nims, R. G., Conner, E. H., Botelho, S. Y. and Comroe, J. H., Jr.: Comparison of methods for performing manual artificial respiration on apneic patients, J. Appl Physiol 4:486, 1951.

62. Dripps, R. D.: Medicine of the Year—Anesthesiology Section, Philadelphia, J. B. Lippincott, 1951.

63. King, B. D., Harris, L. C., Jr. and Greifenstein, F. E.: Cardiovascular effects of orotracheal intubation during light anesthesia, Surgical Forum, Anesthesiology, Philadelphia, W. B. Saunders, 1951, p. 620.

64. Eckenhoff, J. E. and Comroe, J. H., Jr.: Blocking action of tetraethylammonium on lobelin-induced thoracic pain. (18608), Proc Soc Exp Biol Med 76:725, 1951.

65. Eckenhoff, J. E., Elder, J. D. and King, B. D.: N-allyl-nor-morphine in the treatment of morphine or demerol narcosis, Am J Med Sci 223:191, 1952.

66. Price, H. L., Conner, E. H., Elder, J. D. and Dripps, R. D.: Effect of sodium thiopental on circulatory response to positive pressure inflation of lung, J Appl Physiol 4:629, 1952.

67. Greifenstein, F. E., King, R. M., Latch, S. S. and Comroe, J. H.: Pulmonary function studies in healthy men and women 50 years and older, J Appl Physiol 4:641, 1952.

68. Elder, J. D., Barker, H. G. and Walker, J. M.: Effect of oxypolygelatin, plasma and 0.9% sodium chloride solution on plasma volume of human subjects after hemorrhage, Fed Proc 11: March, 1952.

69. Vandam, L. D.: The functional anatomy of the lung, Anesthesiology 13:130, 1952.

70. King, B. D., Sokoloff, L. and Wechsler, R. L.: The effects of 1-epinephrine and 1-nor-epinephrine upon cerebral circulation and metabolism in man, J Clin Invest 31:273, 1952.

78

71. Dripps, R. D.: The anesthetic management of the "poor-risk" patient, Bull Ayer Clin Lab *4:*93, 1952.

72. Eckenhoff, J. E., Hoffman, G. L. and Dripps, R. D.: N-allyl normorphine: An antagonist to the opiates, Anesthesiology *13:*242, 1952.

73. King, B. D., Elder, J. D. and Dripps, R. D.: The effect of the intravenous administration of meperidine upon the circulation of man and upon the circulatory response to tilt, Surg Gynec Obstet *94:*591, 1952.

74. Dripps, R. D. and Vandam, L. D.: The anesthetic management of patients with heart disease, Circulation *5:*927, 1952.

75. Barker, H. G., Elder, J. D., Walker, J. M. and Vars, H. M.: An evaluation of methods for comparing plasma volume expanders in man, Surgical Forum, American College of Surgeons, Philadelphia, W. B. Saunders, 1952.

76. Dripps, R. D.: Medicine of the Year—Anesthesiology Section, Philadelphia, J. B. Lippincott, 1952, p. 89.

77. Price, H. L., Conner, E. H. and Dripps, R. D.: Concerning the increase in central venous and arterial blood pressures during cyclopropane anesthesia in man, Anesthesiology *14:*1, 1953.

78. Dripps, R. D.: Abnormal respiratory responses to various "curare" drugs during surgical anesthesia: Incidence, etiology, and treatment, Ann Surg *137:*145, 1953.

79. Price, H. L. and Conner, E. H.: Certain aspects of the hemodynamic response to the Valsalva maneuver, J Appl Physiol *5:*449, 1953.

80. Blakemore, W. S., Dumke, P. R. and Rhoads, J. E.: Gangrene following intra-arterial transfusion, JAMA *151:*988, 1953.

81. Vandam, L. D., Safar, P. and Dumke, P. R.: A new antagonist to Syncurine, Curr Res Anesth Analg *32:*113, 1953.

82. Eckenhoff, J. E.: Preanesthetic sedation of children, Arch Otolaryng (Chicago) *57:*411, 1953.

83. Dripps, R. D.: Anesthesia for the battle casualty. Postgraduate Course on Recent Advances in Medicine of Military Importance, Army Med Service Graduate School, Walter Reed Army Med Center, Washington, DC, May 7, 1953.

84. Zindler, M. and Deming, M. van N.: The anesthetic management of infants for the surgical repair of congenital atresia of the esophagus with tracheoesophageal fistula, Curr Res Anesth Analg *32:*180, 1953.

85. Eckenhoff, J. E., Hoffman, G. L. and Funderburg, L. W.: N-Allylnormorphine: An antagonist to neonatal narcosis produced by sedation of the parturient, Am J Obst Gynec *65:*1269, 1953.

86. Severinghaus, J. W.: A device whereby a circle rebreathing system may be instantaneously interchanged with a non-rebreathing system, Anesthesiology *14:*413, 1953.

87. Nims, R. G., Severinghaus, J. W. and Comroe, J. H.: Reflex hyperpnea induced by papaverine acting upon the carotid and aortic bodies, J Pharmacol Exp Ther *109:*58, 1953.

88. Dripps, R. D.: Cardio-respiratory problems during thoracic operation. Symposium on Circulation and Homeostasis, Army Med Service Graduate School, Walter Reed Army Med Center, Washington, DC, October 7, 1953.

89. Eckenhoff, J. E.: Relationship of anesthesia to postoperative personality changes in children, Am J Dis Child *86:*587, 1953.

90. Dripps, R. D.: The toxic and metabolic effects of general anesthetic agents on the central nervous system, Met Tox Dis Nerv Sys 32:432, 1953.

91. Eckenhoff, J. E., Helrich, M. and Hege, M. J. D.: The effects of narcotics upon the respiratory response to carbon dioxide in man, Surgical Forum, Anesthesiology, Philadelphia, W. B. Saunders, 1953, p. 681.

92. Dripps, R. D.: Medicine of the Year—Anesthesiology Section, Philadelphia, J. B. Lippincott, 1953.

93. Bartels, J., Severinghaus, J. W., Forster, R. E., Briscoe, W. A. and Bates, D. V.: The respiratory dead space measured by single breath analysis of oxygen, carbon dioxide, nitrogen or helium, J Clin Invest 33:41, 1954.

94. Vandam, L. D. and Eckenhoff, J. E.: The anesthesiologist and therapeutic nerve block: technician or physician, Anesthesiology 15:89, 1954.

95. Peterson, L. H., Helrich, M., Greene, L. and Taylor, C.: Measurement of cardiac output: a new method. Fed Proc 13:368, 1954.

96. Peterson, L. H.: The dynamics of pulsatile blood flow, Circ Res 2:127, 1954.

97. Price, H. L., Conner, E. H. and Dripps, R. D.: Some respiratory and circulatory effects of mechanical respirators, J Appl Physiol 6:517, 1954.

98. Dripps, R. D.: Anesthesia for combat casualties on the basis of experience in Korea. Course on Recent Advances in Med and Surg, Army Med Service Graduate School, Walter Reed Army Med Center, Washington, DC, April 19, 1954.

99. King, B. D., Elder, J. D. Proctor, D. F. and Dripps, R. D.: Reflex circulatory responses to tracheal intubation performed under topical anesthesia, Anesthesiology 15:231, 1954.

100. Vitale, A., Dumke, P. R. and Comroe, J. H.: Lack of correlation between rales and arterial oxygen saturation in patients with pulmonary congestion and edema, Circulation 10:81, 1954.

101. Eckenhoff, J. E., Helrich, M, and Hege, M. J. D.: The effects of narcotics upon the respiratory response to carbon dioxide in man, Am J Med Sci 228:3, 1954.

102. Severinghaus, J. W.: The rate of uptake of nitrous oxide in man, J Clin Invest 33:1183, 1954.

103. Dripps, R. D.: The balance sheet on blood transfusion in surgery. Presented at the 5th International Congress of Blood Transfusion, Paris, France, September 15, 1954.

104. Peterson, L. H., Helrich, M., Greene, L., Taylor, D. and Choquette, G.: Measurement of left ventricular output, J Appl Physiol 7:258, 1954.

105. Eckenhoff, J. E. and Funderburg, L. W.: Observations on the use of the opiate antagonists nalorphine and levallorphan, Am J Med Sci 228:546, 1954.

106. Eckenhoff, J. E. and Dripps, R. D.: The use of norepinephrine in various states of shock, Anesthesiology 15:681, 1954.

107. Peterson, L. H., Greene, L. and Taylor, C.: Certain limitations of circulatory studies utilizing indicator dilution, Am J Physiol 179:3, 1954.

108. Dripps, R. D. and Vandam, L. D.: Long-term follow-up of patients who received 10,098 spinal anesthetics. Failure to discover major neurological sequelae, JAMA 156:1486, 1954.

109. Dripps, R. D.: Anesthesia, Ann Rev Med 5:305, 1954.

110. Vandam, L. D. and Dripps, R. D.: The anesthetic properties of cyclobutane, Anesthesiology 16:48, 1955.

111. Peterson, L. H. and Shepard, R. B.: In vivo determination of arterial distensibility and viscous resistance in dogs, Fed Proc *14:*370, 1955.

112. Shepard, R. B. and Peterson, L. H.: Model studies in pressure pulse formation, Fed Proc *14:*448, 1955.

113. Eckenhoff, J. E., Helrich, M., Hege, M. J. D. and Jones, R. E.: The combination of opiate antagonists and opiates for the prevention of respiratory depression, J. Pharmacol Exp Ther *113:*332, 1955.

114. Spencer, R. W., Scheie, H. G. and Dripps, R. D: Anterior chamber injection in the rabbit as a method for determining irritancy of local anesthetics, J Pharmacol Exp Ther *113:*421, 1955.

115. Oech, S. R.: A cuffed endotracheal tube with an incorporated endobronchial blocker, Anesthesiology *16:*468, 1955.

116. Nims, R. G., Conner, E. H. and Comroe, J. H.: The compliance of the human thorax in anesthetized patients, J Clin Invest *34:*744, 1955.

117. Dripps, R. D.: Hypothermia and artificial hibernation, Henry Ford Hosp Med Bull *3:*57, 1955.

118. Vandam, L. D. and Dripps, R. D.: A long-term follow-up of 10,098 spinal anesthetics. II. Incidence and analysis of minor sensory neurological defects, Surgery *38:*463, 1955.

119. Antonetti, J., Ottolenghi, R. and Dripps, R. D.: Use of a succinylcholine extender, Anesthesiology *16:*742, 1955.

120. Dripps, R. D.: Sedation, analgesia and anesthesia for mass casualties. Management of Mass Casualties Pub No. 570, Walter Reed Army Institute of Res, Washington, DC, September, 1955.

121. Price, H. L. and Helrich, M.: Significance of the compentence index in the measurement of myocardial contractility, J Pharmacol Exp Ther *115:*199, 1955.

122. Price, H. L. and Helrich, M.: The effect of cyclopropane, diethyl ether, nitrous oxide, thiopental, and hydrogen ion concentration on the myocardial function of the dog heart-lung preparation, J Pharmacol Exp Ther *115:*206, 1955.

123. Dripps, R. D. and Severinghaus, J. W.: General anesthesia and respiration, Physiol Rev *35:*741, 1955.

124. Dripps, R. D., Vandam, L. D., Pierce, E. C., Oech, S. R. and Lurie, A. A.: The use of chloropromazine in anesthesia and surgery, Ann Surg *142:*774, 1955.

125. Millar, R. A.: Adrenaline and noradrenaline, Brit J Anaesth 27:603, 1955.

126. Eckenhoff, J. E., Helrich, M., Hege, M. J. D. and Jones, R. E.: Respiratory hazards of opiates and other narcotic analgesics, Surg Gynec Obstet *101:*701, 1955.

127. Dripps, R. D.: Physiological problems in anesthesia related to induced hypothermia, Surg Clin N Am *35:*1573, 1955.

128. Eckenhoff, J. E.: The use of controlled hypotension for surgical procedures, Surg Clin N Am *35:*1579, 1955.

129. Peterson, L. H. and Shepard, R. B.: Some relationships of blood pressure to the cardiovascular system, Surg Clin N Am *35:*1613, 1955.

130. Ravdin, I. S. and Eckenhoff, J. E.: Shock *in* F. Christopher, ed.: Textbook of Surgery, Philadelphia, W. B. Saunders, 1955, pp. 100–108.

131. Royster, H. P. and Ditzler, J. W.: The use of controlled hypotension in operations on the head and neck, Plast Reconstr Surg *17:*9, 1956.

132. Eckenhoff, J. E., Helrich, M. and Hege, M. J. D.: A method for studying respiratory function in awake or anesthetized patients, Anesthesiology *17:*66, 1956.

133. Price, H. L., Helrich, M. and Conner, E. H.: A relation between hemodynamic and plasma volume alterations during general anesthesia in man, J Clin Invest 35:125, 1956.

134. Ditzler, J. W. and Eckenhoff, J. E.: A Comparison of blood loss and operative time in certain surgical procedures completed with and without controlled hypotension, Ann Surg 143:289, 1956.

135. Price, H. L. and Price, M. L.: Determination of diethyl ether in blood, Anesthesiology 17:293, 1956.

136. Jones, R. E., Helrich, M. and Eckenhoff, J. E.: Effects of common respiratory phenomena during general anesthesia on arterial blood pressure and pulse, Anesthesiology 17:325, 1956.

137. DiGiovanni, A. J. and Dripps, R. D.: Abnormal motor movements during divinyl ether anesthesia, Anesthesiology 17:353, 1956.

138. Dripps, R. D.: Sedation, analgesia and anesthesia for mass casualties, Milit Med 118:369, 1956.

139. Helrich, M., Eckenhoff, J. E., Jones, R. E. and Rolph, W. D.: Influence of opiates on the respiratory response of man to thiopental, Anesthesiology 17:459, 1956.

140. Eckenhoff, J. E. and Dam, W.: The treatment of barbiturate poisoning with or without analeptics, Am J Med 20:912, 1956.

141. Vandam, L. D. and Dripps, R. D.: Long-term follow-up of patients who received 10,098 spinal anesthetics. Syndrome of decreased intracranial pressure (headache and ocular and auditory difficulties), JAMA 161:586, 1956.

142. Eckenhoff, J. E.: The anesthesiologist and the management of pain, J Chronic Dis 4:96, 1956.

143. Dundee, J. W., Price, H. L. and Dripps, R. D.: Acute tolerance to thiopentone in man, Brit J Anaesth 28:344, 1956.

144. Valk, A. de T. and Price, H. L.: The chemical estimation of epinephrine and norepinephrine in human and canine plasma. I. A critique of the ethylenediamine condensation method, J Clin Invest 35:837, 1956.

145. Vandam, L. D. and Dripps, R. D.: Exacerbation of pre-existing neurologic disease after spinal anesthesia, New Eng J Med 255:843, 1956.

146. Millar, R. A.: The fluorimetric estimation of epinephrine in peripheral venous plasma during insulin hypoglycemia, J Pharmacol Exp Ther 118:435, 1956.

147. Eckenhoff, J. E.: Some preoperative warnings of potential operating-room deaths, New Eng J Med 255:1075, 1956.

148. Dripps, R. D.: Anesthesia, chap. 12, in Surgery: Principles and Practice, Philadelphia, J. B. Lippincott, 1956.

149. Dundee, J. W., Linde, H. W. and Dripps, R. D.: Observations on trifluoroethylvinyl ether, Anesthesiology 18:66, 1957.

150. Price, H. L., Dundee, J. W. and Conner, E. H.: Rates of uptake and release of thiopental by human brain; relation to kinetics of thiopental anesthesia, Anesthesiology 18:171, 1957.

151. Dundee, J. W. and Dripps, R. D.: Effects of diethyl ether, trichloroethylene and trifluoroethylvinyl ether on respiration, Anesthesiology 18:282, 1957.

152. Price, H. L.: Circulating adrenaline and noradrenaline during diethyl ether anaesthesia in man, Clin Sci 16:377, 1957.

153. Kraft, W. F., Wolff, R. C. and Eckenhoff, J. E.: A comparison of the sedative effects of chloral hydrate, ethinimate and pentobarbital in man, Anesth Analg (Cleveland) 36:44, 1957.

154. Dripps, R. D., Millar, R. A. and Kneale, D. H.: A comparison of anileridine, morphine and meperidine in man, Surg Gynec Obstet *105:*322, 1957.

155. Eckenhoff, J. E., Helrich, M. and Rolph, W. D.: The effects of promethazine upon respiration and circulation of man, Anesthesiology *18:*703, 1957.

156. Eckenhoff, J. E.: Anesthesia and operation for the patient with heart disease, J Kentucky Med Ass *55:*887, 1957.

157. Dripps, R. D.: Hazards of the immediate postoperative period, JAMA *165:*795, 1957.

158. Price, H. L. and Price, M. L.: The chemical estimation of epinephrine and norepinephrine in human and canine plasma. II. A critique of the trihydroxyindole method, J Lab Clin Med *50:*769, 1957.

159. Eckenhoff, J. E., Helrich, M. and Rolph, W. D.: The effect of dihydrocodeine upon respiration and circulation in man, Anesthesiology *18:*891, 1957.

160. Eckenhoff, J. E.: Opiate poisoning, *in* Howard B. Conn, ed.: Current Therapy for 1958, Philadelphia, W. B. Saunders.

161. Price, H. L., Lurie, A. A., Jones, R. E. and Linde, H. W.: Role of catecholamines in the initiation of arrhythmic cardiac contraction by carbon dioxide inhalation in anesthetized man, J Pharmacol Exp Ther *122:*7885, 1958.

162. Dripps, R. D.: The physician's responsibilities toward blood transfusions, Southern Med J *51:*141, 1958.

163. Eckenhoff, J. E. and Norton, M. L.: The treatment of intractable pain with large doses of morphine and amiphenazole (Daptazole), Acta Anaesth Scand *2:*45, 1958.

164. Price, H, L., Price, M. L. and Jones, R. E.: Norepinephrinemia during diethyl ether and cyclopropane anesthesia in man, Fed Proc *17:*498, 1958.

165. Eckenhoff, J. E. and Helrich, M.: The effect of narcotics, thiopental and nitrous oxide upon respiration and respiratory response to hypercapnia, Anesthesiology *19:*240, 1958.

166. Eckenhoff, J. E.: The physiology of hypothermia, Bull NY Acad Med *34:*297, 1958.

167. Eckenhoff, J. E. and Helrich, M.: Study of narcotics and sedatives for use in preanesthetic medication, JAMA *167:*415, 1958.

168. Sechzer, P. H.: Effect of hypothermia on compliance and resistance of the lung-thorax system of anesthetized man, J Appl Physiol *13:*53, 1958.

169. Zaimis, E., Cannard, T. H. and Price, H. L.: Effects of lowered muscle temperature upon neuromuscular blockade in man, Science *128:*34, 1958.

170. Eckenhoff, J. E.: An author's best friend (editorial), Anesthesiology *19:*554, 1958.

171. Lurie, A. A., Jones, R. E., Linde, H. W., Price, M. L., Dripps, R. D. and Price, H. L.: Cyclopropane anesthesia. I. Cardiac rate and rhythm during steady levels of cyclopropane anesthesia at normal and elevated end-expiratory carbon dioxide tensions, Anesthesiology *19:*457, 1958.

172. Egbert, L. D., Norton, M. L., Eckenhoff, J. E. and Dripps, R. D.: A comparison in man of the effects of promethazine, secobarbital, and meperidine alone and in combination on certain respiratory functions and for use in preanesthetic medication, Southern Med J *51:*1173, 1958.

173. Price, H. L., Lurie, A. A., Jones, R. E., Price, M. L. and Linde, H. W.: Cyclopropane anesthesia. II. Epinephrine and norepinephrine in initiation of ventricular arrhythmias by carbon dioxide inhalation, Anesthesiology *19:*619, 1958.

174. Egbert, L. D., Sechzer, P. H. and Eckenhoff, J. E.: Comparative hypnosis produced by methitural (Neraval) and thiopental, Anesthesiology 19:656, 1958.
175. Oech. S. R. and Dripps, R. D.: Judgment in anesthesia, Surg Clin N Am, October, 1958, p. 1205.
176. Linde, H. W. and Price, H. L.: Gas analyzer for rapid estimation of cyclopropane, Anesthesiology 19:757, 1958.
177. Linde, H. W. and Lurie, A. A.: Infrared analysis for carbon dioxide in respired gases containing cyclopropane and ether, Anesthesiology 20:45, 1959.
178. Cannard, T. H. and Schuder, J. C.: A simple operating room electro-cardiogram monitor, Surgery 45:467, 1959.
179. Dripps, R. D.: Use of monitoring devices during anesthesia and operation, Perspect Biol Med 2:362, 1959.
180. Price, H. L. and Conner, E. H.: Rate of uptake of thiopental by body fat; its relation to the duration of narcosis, Fed Proc 18:1714, 1959.
181. Egbert, L. D., Dumas, P. A., Ginter, G. C. and Eckenhoff, J. E.: Modification of the circulatory response to electroshock therapy by thiopental, Anesthesiology 20:309, 1959.
182. Eckenhoff, J. E.: Phenazocine, a new benzomorphan narcotic analgesic, Anesthesiology 20:355, 1959.
183. Cannard, T. H.: Adaptors for ECG electrodes, Anesthesiology 20:383, 1959.
184. Price, H. L.: Estimation of epinephrine and norepinephrine concentrations in human plasma by the trihydroxyindole method, Pharmacol Rev 11:273, 1959.
185. Black, G. W., Linde, H. W., Dripps, R. D. and Price, H. L.: Circulatory changes accompanying respiratory acidosis during halothane (Fluothane) anaesthesia in man, Brit J Anaesth 31:238, 1959.
186. Eckenhoff, J. E.: Introduction, a symposium on muscle relaxants, Anesthesiology 20:407, 1959.
187. Dripps, R. D.: The role of muscle relaxants in anesthesia deaths, Anesthesiology 20:542, 1959.
188. Price, H. L., Linde, H. W., Jones, R. E., Black, G. W. and Price, M. L.: Sympatho-adrenal responses to general anesthesia in man and their relation to hemodynamics, Anesthesiology 20:563, 1959.
189. Dripps, R. D., Hanks, E. C., Ngai, S. H., Oech. S. R., Papper, E. M. and Sechzer, P. H.: A clinical study of the muscle relaxant—Imbretil, Anesthesiology 20:646, 1959.
190. Eckenhoff, J. E.: What you read (editorial), Anesthesiology 20:698, 1959.
191. Egbert, L. D., Oech, S. R. and Eckenhoff, J. E.: Comparison of the recovery from methohexital and thiopental anesthesia in man, Surg Gynec Obstet 109:427, 1959.
192. Dripps, R. D., Linden, M. E., Morris, H. H. and Phillips, W. A.: Medical, social and legal aspects of suicide, JAMA 171:523, 1959.
193. Eckenhoff, J. E.: Postanesthetic respiratory depression, Texas J Med 55:797, 1959.
194. Sechzer, P. H., Dripps, R. D. and Price, H. L.: Uptake of cyclopropane by the human body, J Appl Physiol 14:887, 1959.
195. Linde, H. W.: Gas analysis by thermal conductivity, Anesthesiology 20:884, 1959
196. Cannard, T. H. and Zaimis, E.: The effect of lowered muscle temperature on the action of neuromuscular blocking drugs in man, J Physiol 149:112, 1959.

84

Bibliography 1943 to 1965

197. Eckenhoff, J. E.: Opiate poisoning, *in* Howard B. Conn, ed.: Current Therapy for 1959, Philadelphia, W. B. Saunders, 1959, p. 682.

198. Eckenhoff, J. E.: The Anesthesia Memorial Foundation (editorial), Anesthesiology *21:*78, 1960.

199. Price, H. L., Kovnat, P. J., Safer, J. N., Conner, E. H. and Price, M. L.: The uptake of thiopental by body tissues and its relation to the duration of narcosis, Clin Pharmacol Ther *1:*16, 1960.

200. Price, H. L.: A dynamic concept of the distribution of thiopental in the human body, Anesthesiology *21:*40, 1960.

201. Craythorne, N. W. B., Rottenstein, H. S. and Dripps, R. D.: The effect of succinylcholine on intraocular pressure in adults, infants and children during general anesthesia, Anesthesiology *21:*59, 1960.

202. Atkinson, R. S.: Trichlorethylene anesthesia, Anesthesiology *21:*67, 1960.

203. Cannard, T. H., Dripps, R. D., Helwig, J. and Zinsser, H. F.: The electrocardiogram during anesthesia and surgery, Anesthesiology *21:*194, 1960.

204. Price, H. L. and Price, M. L.: Simplification of method for determination of ether, Anesthesiology *21:*222, 1960.

205. Vandam, L. D. and Dripps, R. D.: Long-term follow-up of patients who received 10,098 spinal anesthetics. IV. Neurological disease incident to traumatic lumbar puncture during spinal anesthesia, JAMA *172:*1483, 1960.

206. Price, H. L.: General anesthesia and circulatory homeostasis, Physiol Rev *40:*187, 1960.

207. Sechzer, P. J., Egbert, L. D., Linde, H. W., Cooper, D. Y., Dripps, R. D. and Price, H. L.: Effect of CO_2 inhalation on arterial pressure, ECG and plasma catecholamines and 17-OH corticosteroids in normal man, J Appl Physiol *15:*454, 1960.

208. Price, H. L., Linde, H. W. and Price, M. L.: Failure of ethylenediamine condensation method to detect increased plasma norepinephrine concentrations during general anesthesia in man, Clin Pharmacol Ther *1:*298, 1960.

209. Prevoznik, S. J. and Eckenhoff, J. E.: The use of phenazocine (Prinadol) in surgical patients, Surg Gynec Obstet *110:*669, 1960.

210. Schuder, J. C., Cannard, T. H., Aiken, D. W., Bouzoukis, J. K. and Kirby, C. K.: EEG electrode burns associated with simultaneous use of electrocautery: cause and prevention, Trans ASAIG *6:*355, 1960.

211. Prockop, L. D., Eckenhoff, J. E. and McElroy, R. C.: Evaluation of dextropropoxyphene, codeine, and acetylsalicylic compound, Obstet Gynec *16:*113, 1960.

212. Jones, R. E., Guldmann, N., Linde, H. W., Dripps, R. D. and Price, H. L.: Cyclopropane anesthesia. III. Effects of cyclopropane on respiration and circulation in normal man, Anesthesiology *21:*380, 1960.

213. Eckenhoff, J. E. and Oech, S. R.: The effects of narcotics and antagonists upon respiration and circulation in man, Clin Pharmacol Ther *1:*483, 1960.

214. Eckenhoff, J. E.: Management of pain, *in* Curtis P. Artz and James D. Hardy, eds.: Complications in Surgery and Their Management, chap. 17, Philadelphia, W. B. Saunders, 1960, pp. 315–323.

215. Craythorne, N. W. B., Turndorf, H. and Dripps, R. D.: Changes in pulse rate and rhythm associated with the use of succinylcholine in anesthetized children, Anesthesiology *21:*465, 1960.

216. Wollman, H. and Cannard, T. H.: Skeletal muscle, esophageal and rectal temperatures in man during general anesthesia and operation, Anesthesiology *21:*652, 1960.

217. Price, H. L.: Effects of carbon dioxide on the cardiovascular system, Anesthesiology *21:652*, 1960.

218. Price, H. L., Lurie, A. A., Black, G. W., Sechzer, P. H., Linde, H. W. and Price, M. L.: Modification by general anesthetics (cyclopropane and halothane) of circulatory and sympathoadrenal responses to respiratory acidosis, Ann Surg *152:*1071, 1960.

219. Dripps, R. D.: What is the significance of hypercarbia or hypocarbia in the anesthetized patient? Anesthesiology *21:759*, 1960.

220. Eckenhoff, J. E.: The Choice of a Medical Career, *in* Joseph Garland and Joseph Stokes, III, eds.: Anesthesiology, chap. 16, Philadelphia, J. B. Lippincott, 1961, pp. 167–179.

221. ———: Opiate poisoning, *in* Howard B. Conn, ed.: Current Therapy for 1961, Philadelphia, W. B. Saunders, 1961, pp. 675–677.

222. Jones, R. E., Deutsch, S. and Turndorf, H: Effects of atropine on cardiac rhythm in conscious and anesthetized man, Anesthesiology *22:67*, 1961.

223. Price, H. L.: Circulatory actions of general anesthetic agents and the homeostatic roles of epinephrine and norepinephrine in man, Clin Pharmacol Ther *2:163*, 1961.

224. Eckenhoff, J. E.: Anesthesia and the levels of consciousness, Anesthesiology *22:315*, 1961.

225. Dripps, R. D.: Anesthesia and shock, Fed Proc *20:224*, 1961.

226. Dripps, R. D., Eckenhoff, J. E. and Vandam, L. D.: Introduction to Anesthesia, 2nd ed., Philadelphia, W. B. Saunders, 1961.

227. Eckenhoff, J. E., Kneale, D. H. and Dripps, R. D.: The incidence and etiology of postanesthetic excitement—a clinical survey, Anesthesiology *22:667*, 1961.

228. Dripps, R. D., Lamont, A. and Eckenhoff, J. E.: The role of anesthesia in surgical mortality, JAMA *178:261–266*, 1961.

229. Deming, M. V. and Oech, S. R.: Steroid and antihistaminic therapy for post intubation subglottic edema in infants and children, Anesthesiology *22:933–936*, 1961.

230. Williams, C. H., Deutsch, S., Linde, H. W., Bullough, J. W. and Dripps, R. D.: Effects of intravenously administered succinyldicholine on cardiac rate, rhythm, and arterial blood pressure in anesthetized man, Anesthesiology *22:947–954*, 1961.

231. Eckenhoff, J. E.: Opiate poisoning, *in* Howard P. Conn, ed.: Current Therapy for 1962, Philadelphia, W. B. Saunders, 1962, pp. 661–663.

232. Price, M. L. and Price, H. L.: Effects of general anesthetics on contractile responses of rabbit aortic strips, Anesthesiology *23:16–20*, 1962.

233. Sechzer, P. H., Linde, H. W. and Dripps, R. D.: Uptake of halothane by the human body. (Work in Progress abstract), Anesthesiology *23:161–162*, 1962.

234. Price, H. L. and Widdicombe, J.: Actions of cyclopropane on carotid sinus baroreceptors and carotid body chemoreceptors, J Pharmacol Exp Ther *135:233–239*, 1962.

235. Deutsch, S., Linde, H. W. and Price, H. L.: Circulatory and sympathoadrenal responses to cyclopropane in the dog, J Pharmacol Ther *135:354–357*, 1962.

236. Price, H. L., Jones, R. E., Deutsch, S. and Linde, H. W.: Ventricular function and autonomic nervous activity during cyclopropane anesthesia in man, J Clin Invest *41*:604–610, 1962.

237. Dripps, R. D.: Decisions for a specialty, Bull NY Acad Med *38*:264–270, 1962.

238. Jones, R. E., Linde, H. W., Deutsch, S., Dripps, R. D. and Price, H. L.: Hemodynamic actions of diethyl ether in normal man, Anesthesiology *23*:299–305, 1962.

239. Pulver, S. E., Hoffman, G. L. and Sechzer, P. H.: Hypnosis, Am Pract *13*: 274–284, 1962.

240. Eckenhoff, J. E.: The New England Journal of Medicine (editorial), Anesthesiology *23*:386–388, 1962.

241. Pierce, E. C., Lambertsen, C. J., Deutsch, S., Chase, P. E., Linde, H. W., Dripps, R. D. and Price, H. L.: Cerebral circulation and metabolism during thiopental anesthesia and hyperventilation in man, J Clin Invest *41*:1664–1671, 1962.

242. Chance, B., Cohen, P. J., Jobsis, F. and Schoener, B.: Intracellular oxidation-reduction states in vivo, Science *137*:499–508, 1962.

243. Deutsch, S., Linde, H. W., Dripps, R. D. and Price, H. L.: Circulatory and respiratory actions of halothane in normal man, Anesthesiology *23*:631–638, 1962.

244. Dripps, R. D., Lamont, A. and Eckenhoff, J. E.: La part de l'anesthesie dans la mortalite operatoire, Cah Anesth *10*:7–22, 1962.

245. Eckenhoff, J. E.: Observations during hypotensive anaesthesia, Proc Roy Soc Med *55*:942–944, 1962.

246. Forster, R. E., Craw, M. R., Constantine, H. P. and Morello, J. A.: Gas exchange processes in the pulmonary capillaries, *in* A. V. S. de Reuck and Maeve O'Connor, eds.: Ciba Foundation Symposium on Pulmonary Structure and Function, London, J. & A. Churchill Ltd., 1962, pp. 215–228.

247. Price, H. L., Cook, W. A., Deutsch, S., Linde, H. W., Mishalove, R. D. and Morse, H. T.: Hemodynamic and central nervous actions of cyclopropane in the dog, Anesthesiology *24*:1–10, 1963.

248. Dripps, R. D.: Anesthesia in the office and small hospital, Postgrad Med *33*:123–127, 1963.

249. Eckenhoff, J. E.: Opiate poisoning, *in* Howard F. Conn, ed.: Current Therapy for 1963, Philadelphia, W. B. Saunders, 1963, pp. 661–663.

250. Price, H. L., Morse, H. T. and Linde, H. W.: Central nervous actions of halothane which affect the circulation, Anesthesiology *24*:139, 1963.

251. Craw, M. R., Constantine, H. P., Morello, J. A. and Forster, R. E.: Rate of the Bohr shift in human red cell suspensions, J Appl Physiol *18*:317–327, 1963.

252. Morse, H. T., Price, M. L. and Price, H. L.: Effects of halothane on systemic baroreceptors, Fed Proc *22*:187 (#158), March-April, 1963.

253. Eckenhoff, J. E. and Judevine, D. E.: The influence of deliberate hypotension and $P_a CO_2$ on jugular bulb oxygen tensions, Fed Proc *22*:344 (#1100), March-April, 1963.

254. Holderness, M. C., Chase, P. E. and Dripps, R. D.: A narcotic analgesic and a butyrophenone with nitrous oxide for general anesthesia, Anesthesiology *24*:336–340, 1963.

255. Alexander, S. C.: Controlled acid-base status with cardiopulmonary bypass and hypothermia, Anesthesiology *24*:400–402, 1963.

256. Dripps, R. D.: Pharmacology of general anesthetic agents, Science *140:* 1247, 1963.

257. Dripps, R. D., Strong, M. J. and Price, H. L.: The heart and general anesthesia, Mod Conc Cardiov Dis *32:*805–808, 1963.

258. Moore, E. N., Morse, H. T. and Price, H. L.: Cardiac arrhythmias produced by norepinephrine in anesthetized dogs, Physiologist *6:*239 (August), 1963.

259. Price, H. L.: Circulation: general considerations, *in* Uptake and Distribution of Anesthetic Agents, New York, McGraw-Hill, 1963, pp. 123–139.

260. Sechzer, P. H.: Cyclopropane, *in* Uptake and Distribution of Anesthetic Agents, New York, McGraw-Hill, 1963, pp. 265–273.

261. Eckenhoff, J. E.: The care of the unconscious patient, JAMA *186:*541–543, 1963.

262. Dripps, R. D.: Pharmacodynamics of human disease. 2. Therapeutic application of opiates, Postgrad Med *34:*520–524, 1963.

263. Price, H. L., Linde, H. W. and Morse, H. T.: Central nervous actions of halothane affecting the systemic circulation, Anesthesiology *24:*770–778, 1963.

264. Sechzer, P. H., Linde, H. W., Dripps, R. D. and Price, H. L.: Uptake of halothane by the human body, Anesthesiology *24:*779–783, 1963.

265. Morse, H. T., Linde, H. W., Mishalove, R. D. and Price, H. L.: Relation of blood volume and hemodynamic changes during halothane anesthesia in man, Anesthesiology *24:*790–795, 1963.

266. Sechzer, P. H.: Subdural space in spinal anesthesia, Anesthesiology *24:*869–870, 1963.

267. Linde, H. W. and Butler, R. A.: Residue in halothane vaporizer, Anesthesiology *24:*887, 1963.

268. Eckenhoff, J. E., Enderby, G. E. H., Larson, A., Davies, R. and Judevine, D. E.: Human cerebral circulation during deliberate hypotension and head-up tilt J Appl Physiol *18:*1130–1138, 1963.

269. Eckenhoff, J. E., Enderby, G. E. H., Larson, A., Edridge, A. and Judevine, D. E.: Pulmonary gas exchange during deliberate hypotension, Brit J Anaesth *35:* 750–759, 1963.

270. Alexander, S. C., Wollman, H., Cohen, P. J., Chase, P. E., Melman, E. and Behar, M.: Krypton[85] and nitrous oxide uptake of the human brain during anesthesia, Anesthesiology *25:*37–42, 1964.

271. Dripps, R. D.: General anesthesia and the circulation, Proc Am Philosophical Soc *108:*15–18, 1964.

272. Wollman, H., Alexander, S. C., Cohen, P. J., Chase, P. E., Melman, E. and Behar, M. G.: Cerebral circulation of man during halothane anesthesia: Effects of hypocarbia and of d-tubocurarine, Anesthesiology *25:*180–184, 1964.

273. Cohen, P. J., Wollman, H., Alexander, S. C., Chase, P. E. and Behar, M. G.: Cerebral carbohydrate metabolism in man during halothane anesthesia: Effects of $P_a CO_2$ on some aspects of carbohydrate utilization, Anesthesiology *25:*185–191, 1964.

274. Butler, R. A.: Pharmacokinetics of halothane and ether, Brit J Anaesth *36:*193–199, 1964.

275. Askrog, V. F., Pender, J. W., Smith, T. C. and Eckenhoff, J. E.: Changes in respiratory dead space during halothane, cyclopropane, and nitrous oxide anesthesia, Anesthesiology *25:*342–352, 1964.

276. Butler, R. A. and Linde, H. W.: Trace compounds in halothane, Anesthesiology 25:397–398, 1964.

277. Price, H. L. and Cohen, P. J., eds.: Effects of Anesthetics on the Circulation, Springfield (Ill.), Charles C. Thomas, 1964.

278. Wollman, H.: The cerebral circulation during halothane anesthesia, chap. 12-C, *in* Effects of Anesthetics on the Circulation, Springfield (Ill.), Charles C. Thomas, 1964, pp. 209–215.

279. Moore, E. N., Morse, H. T. and Price, H. L.: Cardiac arrhythmias produced by catecholamines in anesthetized dogs, Circ Res 15:77–82, 1964.

280. Askrog, V. F. and Eckenhoff, J. E.: Intra-arterial blood-pressure recording as a teaching aid in anesthesia, Acta Anaesth Scand 8:131–141, 1964.

281. Eckenhoff, J. E. and Melman, E.: Deliberate hypotension in the control of operative bleeding, Ann NY Acad Sci 115:341–347, July 9, 1964.

282. Dripps, R. D.: Research: The environment for maximal development, Anesthesiology 25:440–444, 1964.

283. Alexander, S. C., Wollman, H., Cohen, P. J., Chase, P. E. and Behar, M.: Cerebrovascular response to $P_a Co_2$ during halothane anesthesia in man, J Appl Physiol 19:561–565, 1964.

284. Askrog, V. F., Smith, T. C. and Eckenhoff, J. E.: Changes in pulmonary ventilation during spinal anesthesia, Surg Gynec Obstet 119:563–567, 1964.

285. Larson, A. G.: Deliberate hypotension, Anesthesiology 25:682–706, 1964.

286. Eckenhoff, J. E., Compton, J. R., Larson, A. and Davies, R. M.: Assessment of cerebral effects of deliberate hypotension by psychological measurements, Lancet 2:711–714, 1964.

287. Dripps, R. D.: The present status of anesthesiology. A survey, Ann Surg 160:640–642, 1964.

288. Askrog, V. F., Pender, J. W. and Eckenhoff, J. E.: Changes in physiological dead space during deliberate hypotension, Anesthesiology 25:744–751, 1964.

289. Prevoznik, S. J. and Eckenhoff, J. E.: Phantom sensations during spinal anesthesia, Anesthesiology 25:767–770, 1964.

290. Eckenhoff, J. E.: The effects of deliberate hypotension upon the circulation and respiration. Proc of the 3rd International Congress of Plastic Surgery; Excerpta Med International Congress Series No. 66, October 1963, pp. 378–383.

291. Price, H. L., Price, M. L. and Morse, H. T.: Effects of cyclopropane, halothane and procaine on the vasomotor "center" of the dog, Anesthesiology 26: 55–60, 1965.

292. Eckenhoff, J. E.: Some observations on deliberate hypotension. Proc of the 3rd World Congress of Anaesthesiologists, vol. 2, Sao Paulo, Brazil, September 20–26, 1964, pp. 13–22.

293. Paymaster, N. J., Wollman, H. and Bachman, L.: Cyclopropane induction to endotracheal ether anaesthesia in infants and children, Brit J Anaesth 37:29–34, 1965.

294. Dripps, R. D.: Human pharmacology of a new inhalational anesthetic agent, *in* F. Zaimis, ed.: Evaluation of New Drugs in Man: Proc of the 2nd International Pharmacological Meet, Prague, Czechoslovakia, August 20–23, 1963, New York, Pergamon Press, 1965, pp. 103–110.

295. Price, H. L., Deutsch, S., Cooperman, L. H., Clement, A. J. and Epstein, R. M.: Splanchnic circulation during cyclopropane anesthesia in normal man, Anesthesiology 26:312–319, 1965.

296. Wollman, H., Alexander, S. C., Cohen, P. J., Smith, T. C., Chase, P. E. and Van der Molen, R. A.: Cerebral circulation during general anesthesia and hyperventilation in man: thiopental induction to nitrous oxide and d-tubocurarine, Anesthesiology 26:329–334, 1965.

297. Constantine, H. P., Craw, M. R. and Forster, R. E.: Rate of the reaction of carbon dioxide with human red blood cells, Am J Physiol 208:801–811, 1965.

298. Alexander, S. C., Cohen, P. J., Wollman, H., Smith, T. C., Reivich, M. and Van der Molen, R. A.: Cerebral carbohydrate metabolism during hypocarbia in man: Studies during nitrous oxide anesthesia, Anesthesiology 26:624–632, 1965.

299. Eckenhoff, J. E.: The anesthetists in Thomas Eakins' "Clinics," Anesthesiology 26:663–666, 1965

300. Eckenhoff, J. E. and Cooperman, L. H.: The clinical application of phenoxybenzamine in shock and vasoconstrictive states, Surg Gynec Obstet 121:483–490, 1965.

301. Braddock, L. I. and Marec, N.: The gas chromatographic analysis of submicrogram quantities of barbiturates using a flame ionization detector, J Gas Chromat 3:274–277, 1965.

302. Bruce, D. L. and Marshall, J. M., Jr.: Some ionic and bioelectric properties of the ameba Chaos chaos, J. Gen Physiol 49:151, (September, Part 1), 1965.

303. Brunner, E. A. and Haugaard, N: The effect of thiopental on hepatic glycogen phosphorylase, J Pharmacol Exp Ther 150:99–104, 1965.

304. Dripps, R. D.: Anesthesia, chap. 11, in Moyer, Rhoads, Allen, and Harkins, eds: Surgery: Principles and Practice, 3rd ed., Philadelphia, J. B. Lippincott, 1965, pp. 230–256.

305. Eckenhoff, J. E., ed.: Science and Practice in Anesthesia, Philadelphia, J. B. Lippincott, 1965.

306. Dripps, R. D., Cohen, P. J., Price, H. L. and Wollman, H.: in L. S. Goodman and A. Gilman, eds.: The Pharmacological Basis of Therapeutics, 3rd ed., New York, The Macmillan Co., 1965.

307. Sechzer, P. H.: The effect of organophosphates on nerve conduction. Arch Int Pharmacodyn 157:432–441 (October), 1965.

308. Wollman, H., Alexander, S. C., Cohen, P. J., Stephen, G. W. and Zeiger, L. S.: Two-compartment analysis of the blood flow in the human brain, Acta Neurol Scand 41: (Suppl. 14), 79–82, 1965.

309. Eckenhoff, J. E.: A technic of deliberate hypotension, Anesth Analg (Cleveland) 44:791, 1965.

Indexes

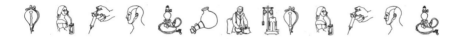

IN THIS BORDER, used in *Anesthesia from Colonial Times* with the kind permission of Leroy D. Vandam, MD, the items represent, left to right,

1. Leroy's "safety" bellows for resuscitation (1827)
2. John Snow's chloroform inhaler
3. Manner of holding syringe while injecting. After Labat
4. Distribution of sensory branches of trigeminal nerve. After Labat
5. Squire's inhaler for ether, first used on 21 December, 1846, by Robert Liston at University College Hospital, London
6. W. T. G. Morton's ether inhaler (1846)
7. J. T. Clover filling reservoir bag (shown over his shoulder) of his chloroform apparatus with a mixture of 4½% chloroform vapor in air (1862)
8. Hele's governor, to control the flow of nitrous oxide from the gas reservoir to the patient (1873).

INDEX OF PERSONAL NAMES

INDEX OF SUBJECTS

94